# More Postgraduate Tutorials in General Practice

# More Postgraduate Tutorials in General Practice

**Edward Warren** MB ChB, MRCGP, DRCOG
General Practitioner, Chapelgreen, Sheffield
GP Trainer, Barnsley Vocational Training Scheme

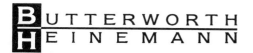

Butterworth-Heinemann Ltd
Linacre House, Jordan Hill, Oxford OX2 8DP

A member of the Reed Elsevier plc group

OXFORD   LONDON   BOSTON
MUNICH   NEW DELHI   SINGAPORE   SYDNEY
TOKYO   TORONTO   WELLINGTON

First edition 1996

© Butterworth-Heinemann Ltd 1996

**British Library Cataloguing in Publication Data**
Warren, W. E.
  More Postgraduate Tutorials in General
  Practice
  I. Title
  362.172

  ISBN 0 7506 2552 X

Filmset by Bath Typesetting Ltd, Bath
Printed and bound in Great Britain by Biddles Ltd, Guildford and King's Lynn

# Contents

# Preface

*Are tutorials useful?*

The tutorial has rather gone out of favour in educational circles, despite its long tradition as a method of medical education. When used as a sort of scaled down lecture where the trainer imparts wisdom to the trainee, the tutorial is a very poor way of transmitting information. However, there should be times when trainer and trainee have time to sit and discuss a relevant topic, and if this time is used properly then much satisfaction can be derived.

Some topics are better dealt with in a tutorial setting. These would include topics where there has been or continues to be some controversy. For others there may be a lot of new information emerging from the literature which has to be assessed and assimilated before it can be used in clinical practice. Yet other issues are more of an ethical or even philosophical nature, and may not appear as issues in the trainee's day to day experience but are important nonetheless.

The trainee's work in the practice will throw up problems, at least from time to time. In the course of a busy surgery with the patient sitting in the consulting room waiting for an answer, it is inappropriate to discuss these problems in depth as what the trainee and the patient will want is an answer with as short a delay as possible.

The trainee will not wish to appear a fool in front of the patient (the 'Wally Factor'), when short of an answer to a routine problem. It is important for the trainee and for the service which the practice provides that the trainee be treated as a fully-fledged GP. You can tell the patients that despite being called 'the trainee', they are nonetheless consulting a fully qualified doctor. This assertion is less convincing if the trainee has to keep disappearing for 15 minutes to have a socratic chat with the trainer about a difficulty.

The choice of tutorial topics is best done with regard to any problems which have arisen in the trainees day by day work. Other topics will be chosen because the trainee feels a lack of confidence in an area. There has to be separate time set aside to deal with these topics. The use of 'hot topic' teaching or the abbreviated 10 minute tutorial are quite separate educational areas.

Trainers are required to set aside uninterrupted teaching time for their trainees, and to plan and implement a learning programme. When the Regional Health Authority and their agents come calling on your re-approval visits, they may well require proof that you are doing with your trainee what you say you are doing. Having a regular tutorial slot timetabled into the week, and a list of tutorials undertaken fits the requirement of proof very nicely.

*Using this book*
There should be enough material in each chapter to provoke about an hour's discussion. The chapter should be read beforehand by each of the participants. The content of each chapter seeks to indicate, with justification, what constitutes good practice. Any controversial areas are discussed with arguments for and against. There is a prevailing emphasis on aspects of the topic which most closely affect general practitioners and their work.

This book, with it's companion volume *Postgraduate Tutorials in General Practice*, covers 32 topics. This is more than enough to provide material for a weekly tutorial over a six month trainee attachment.

The tutorial time can be spent in discussing some of the issues raised, or just generally debating the topic. Sometimes the use of an actual case from the trainee's experience helps to focus the discussion on to practical areas. I would not like to think that the material in this book was used in a didactic and dogmatic way, and though I would hope there are not too many errors in the text, I do not think it should be used as a reference book.

*The choice of subjects*
The subjects of the chapters have largely been chosen by my trainees. Despite the differences between trainees in both interests and educational needs, it is remarkable with what regularity the same topics keep being asked for.

All the tutorials have been 'road tested' with my own trainees, and in many cases only appear in this book having been used on many occasions. I can therefore feel confident that the topics are of sufficient interest and relevance to trainees to lead to a suitable discussion. Some major topics are not included, but the reason for this is simply that they have not been asked for.

*Choosing the aims*
Each chapter is preceded by a list of three or four aims for the tutorial. I think it is important to identify beforehand what you hope the trainee will get from the tutorial, as this is often the

stimulus to hold the tutorial in the first place. You will probably not agree with the aims in the text, at least not completely. I hope that there is sufficient material in the text, however, to address a number of other learning needs which may have been identified.

*The choice of references*
Errors and omissions in the text are entirely my responsibility. Where a statistic has been used, I have tried to site a suitable reference for it. Where an opinion or judgement or assessment is not my own (and has been published elsewhere), then I have tried to indicate the source.

I have used mainly secondary sources as references. This is deliberate and reflects my own reading habits and, I would suggest, those of a majority of 'coal face' GPs. In the cases where guidelines have been published by a British authority, I have used this source extensively. The journals cited, with some exceptions, are those most readily available to British general practitioners and trainees, as well as being available in most postgraduate libraries. A number of references are taken from the free medical newspapers in circulation. I suspect that these are the most widely read medical sources of all.

# Acknowledgements

I would like to thank Dr Geoffrey Smaldon at Butterworth-Heinemann for his encouragement throughout the production of this book, and for being one of the few people who replied when I was touting round to find a publisher. The book's reviewers, Drs Mike Cohen, Alex Khot and Andrew Polmear whose comments caused me not a few sleepless nights, should in retrospect be heartily thanked, though there have been times when I didn't much feel like doing so.

The major acknowledgement must, however, be to my long-suffering wife and children. They have tolerated my obsession with this book for the last year or more without being too critical, and have even allowed me to throw bits of paper all over the floor (which is my idea of a filing system) without more than an occasional muffled cry of anguish. Also I have to include something nice about the family in case I want to do it all over again.

E. W.
Shepley

# The general practitioner and raised blood pressure

## Aims

The trainee should:

- Know which patients will benefit from having their blood pressure (BP) lowered.
- Know how to find, assess and follow up the hypertensive patient.
- Be able to counsel a patient on the benefits and drawbacks of treatment for hypertension.

## Why is hypertension important?

Raised BP is an important risk factor for myocardial infarction (MI), stroke (cerebrovascular accident; CVA) and other vascular disease. In 1992 there were 170 000 deaths in the UK because of MI,[1] or about a third of all deaths. There are also 100 000 people who suffer a first stroke each year, and 64 000 deaths due to stroke.[2]

Fifteen per cent of adults in the UK have BP at a level where treatment would be beneficial. Of these, two-thirds have mild hypertension, that is, a diastolic blood pressure (DBP) of 95 to 109 mmHg. Four per cent of the population have a DBP of 110–129 mmHg, and this group has an untreated 2-year mortality of 20%. A total of 0.5% have a DBP over 130 mmHg, and their untreated 2-year mortality is 60%.[3]

Adequate treatment of raised BP could reduce the rate of heart attack by 14%, and the rate of stroke by 40%.[4]

*The Health of the Nation*[5] has set targets for reducing the rates of stroke and heart attack. Bands 2 and 3 of the Health Promotion programme require screening checks to identify hypertension.[6]

Each GP each year prescribes an average of £10 000-worth of drugs to lower BP.[7] The care of hypertension generates about 260 consultations per GP per year.[8]

## How do you measure blood pressure?

The British Hypertension Society made recommendations in 1986.[9] Nearly all the trials on hypertension have followed these guidelines, so the GP should adhere to them if trial results are to be used to justify treatment.

The patient should have been sitting or lying for 3 minutes. The readings sitting and lying should be the same. The arm should be horizontal and supported at the level of the heart, as a dangling arm increases the reading by 10/10 mmHg. The sphygmomanometer bladder should surround 80% of the arm and the bladder width should be at least 40% of the circumference of the arm: the usually supplied 23 cm cuff is inadequate for adults and a 35 or 42 cm for the obese is recommended. If the cuff is too small, the BP reading is higher.

The cuff should be inflated and pressure let out at 2–3 mmHg per second. If air is let out too fast, then the systolic blood pressure (SBP) measurement is lower, and DBP measurement is higher. As a routine the fifth Korotkoff sound should be used to assess DBP as this is the convention used in trials of hypertension. In conditions such as pregnancy when phase V may not be found, phase IV (muffling of sounds) can be used, and its use should be noted.

The equipment should be properly maintained. Aneroid sphygmomanometers tend to read lower with time.

The initial BP reading is always highest, and up to 50% of high readings become normal on rechecking. It is estimated that 20% of patients who are treated for hypertension only have an elevated BP when someone in a white coat wants to measure it – the so-called 'white coat' hypertensives.[7]

Standing BP should be measured as well in patients whose symptoms or drug regime may be associated with a postural fall. The patient should have been standing for 1 minute before the reading is made. If the sitting and standing BPs differ by more than 20/10 mmHg, then this is abnormal and symptoms of postural hypotension may result.

If the difference between the two arms is more than 20/10 mmHg, then there may be an arterial anomaly. The right arm is usually used for measurement, as occasionally there is a consistent but unimportant difference between the two arms. Follow-up readings should all be done using the same arm.

Many of the trials on BP have used the Hawksley random zero sphygmomanometer. This underreads BP by an average 3.5/7.5 mmHg,[10] so that the readings obtained using a conventional sphygmomanometer on the same patient will be higher. There are clear implications about the applicability of the trials to normal practice, and the validity of the meta-analyses done using these trials.

## Ambulatory BP monitoring

All the major trials on hypertension have used 'snapshot' readings of BP taken with a sphygmomanometer. If these trials are to be used to inform treatment of hypertensives, then it makes sense that the same measurement technique should be used.

Ambulatory BP monitoring measures pressure many times over 24 hours, and usually gives lower overall readings than the 'snapshot' approach. In particular, there is usually a 20% fall in BP during sleep. The absence of this fall is associated with secondary causes of hypertension, and with an increased risk of left ventricular hypertrophy.[11]

Ambulatory monitoring is also a good way of selecting out the 'white coat' hypertensives. Whereas 20% of patients with a DBP under 105 mmHg on testing fall into the 'white coat' category, this falls to under 5% in those with a DBP of over 105 mmHg,[12] and this is a group of patients who will almost certainly benefit from treatment.

## Who should have their blood pressure measured?

In their much-quoted paper, Wilson and Jungner[13] gave criteria for screening which have been widely adopted. The condition being screened for must be important, with a recognizable early stage, and early treatment must be of benefit. A suitable test must be available which is acceptable to the population being screened. There must be sufficient resources for treatment, and treatment must be cost-effective. A population to be screened and the frequency of the screening test must be agreed.

Screening the population for raised BP is justified:

- Hypertension is usually asymptomatic and so can only be detected by measurement.
- Hypertension is common among the adult population of the UK. Hypertension is a known risk factor for a number of important diseases, including MI and CVA.
- Treatment of hypertension is known to improve morbidity and mortality.

Opportunistic screening for hypertension is recommended, and this is reinforced by the financial rewards available to GPs who get to band 2 or beyond of the Health Promotion targets. To achieve this, each year an increasing percentage of the practice list are required to have had their BP measured. In the course of a year the GP will see around 70% of patients on the list, and 90% over 3 years. Older patients will in general be seen more frequently. These consultations for other reasons provide an ideal opportunity for BP screening.

GPs who are trying to fulfil the requirements of the Health Promotion bands will have developed a call and recall system for 'well person' checks on the patients who have not consulted recently. This job may well be entrusted to the practice nursing team, and a formal protocol for the checks should include a measure of the BP with provision for follow-up and referral to the GP where appropriate.

The target ages for the health promotion bands are 15–75 years. There is little evidence that the routine screening of children is justified,[14] but benefits in the elderly can be seen at least to age 80.[15] It may be concluded that all people between 15 and 80 should have had their BP measured in the previous 5 years.

It has been estimated that the rule of halves applies to hypertension:[7]

- Half of hypertensives are known.
- Half of known hypertensives are treated.
- Half of treated hypertensives have their BP under control.

Whether the Health Promotion targets will improve the position is as yet undetermined.

## Does treating hypertension do any good?

Over the past 15 years the results of several major trials on the treatment of hypertension have been published. The benefit of treating very high BP is well-established, but the numbers of patients with these levels of BP is not great.

More emphasis has been put on the treatment of mild hypertension. The risk for each individual patient is small, but there are so many people with this level of BP that the cumulative effect on morbidity and mortality is significant.

Interpretation of the trials is difficult. In its review of the evidence in 1989, the British Hypertension Society noted the following difficulties in interpretation.[16]

## Technical problems

The surveys done have used different populations (some hospital-based), different treatments, different age groups. Some were poorly controlled, some only single-blind, and some had no placebo group when comparing different treatments.

## Confidence limits

The majority of surveys have included 'neutral' within the 95% confidence limits for improvement in overall mortality with treatment.

## Effect on MIs

Nearly all surveys show a decrease in the number of strokes in hypertensives treated but no significant decrease in cardiac morbidity/mortality has been found in any one trial. Evidence for the benefit of treatment to reduce MI has only been extracted by meta-analysis of pooled data.[4]

## At-risk groups

No at-risk subgroups have been found, except that men are more at risk than women (but hypertension is commoner in women), and smoking remains highly significant.

## Regression to the norm

Up to half high BPs return to normal on prolonged observation.

## Tolerance of treatment

There has been a significant drop-out rate in all trials – for instance, it was 40% in the Medical Research Council trial of mild hypertension.[17]

# How can you sort out the evidence?

The risks conferred by raised BP are linearly related to the level of BP. Defining threshold levels for treatment is thus a matter of opinion.

Raised BP is only one of number of risk factors for vascular disease. These factors are additive, so that for an individual the risk of the BP may be small compared with the other risks present. On the other hand, those at high risk have the most to gain from an improvement in any of their risks, so that modifiable factors such as raised BP are particularly important as far as treatment is concerned.

Fortuitously, the path through the minefield has been determined by a series of reports from the British Hypertension Society, the last of which was published in 1993.[15] For the time being, those without the time, interest or inclination to rummage through the evidence themselves can confidently regard these guidelines as the official truth, at least until the next report.

## Recommendations of the British Hypertension Society

Consider a management plan based on a *random BP check in general practice*:

**Diastolic blood pressure**

1. Under 90 mmHg – recheck after 5 years.
2. 90–99 mmHg – recheck each month for 3–6 months. If DBP stays under 100 mmHg, then the decision to treat depends on other factors such as age over 60, male sex, smoking, abnormal lipids, a strong family history of coronary heart disease (CHD), or evidence of end-organ damage or diabetes. Average readings in the upper part of this range may encourage treatment. Twenty per cent of patients with a BP of 160/90 mmHg will over the course of 5 years see this rise to over 200/110 mmHg.[4] A plan for chronic monitoring should be instituted, for instance using patients' birthdays as a reminder that it's time to get their BP checked.
3. 100–109 mmHg – if there is no evidence of end-organ damage or diabetes, then repeat the measurement weekly and thereafter monthly. Institute non-drug treatment. If DBP stays under 100 mmHg, then continue. If average DBP is over 100 mmHg, then the patient will benefit from drug treatment.
4. Over 110 mmHg – Repeat measurements should be made over 1–2 weeks, and if the DBP is confirmed, then treatment is indicated.
5. Over 140 mmHg – this is accelerated or malignant hypertension. Repeat the reading several times at the same visit, and look in the eyes for retinal changes. If the BP level is confirmed, then the patient requires admission.

## Systolic blood pressure

Nearly all the major trials on BP have concentrated on the effects and treatment of DBP. However, SBP is also a risk factor for CVA and CHD. Isolated systolic hypertension is rare in younger patients but not uncommon in the elderly.

1. SBP over 160 mmHg on repeated measurement, and end-organ damage present – then the patient will benefit from treatment.
2. SBP over 160 mmHg and no end-organ damage:
   - SBP over 200 mmHg, or SBP over 160 mmHg and DBP over 95 mmHg – then treatment is beneficial.
   - SBP 160–200 mmHg, and DBP under 95 mmHg – review the patient over 3–6 months and treat if the average SBP is over 160 mmHg.

## How do you assess end-organ damage?

If organ damage due to hypertension is found, the patient is more likely to benefit from treatment, and more likely to need referral to a specialist. An assessment will be necessary in patients with a DBP of over 90 mmHg and/or an SBP of over 160 mmHg.

The main effects of hypertension are on the heart, kidneys and blood vessels. Suitable ways of assessing for damage would be:

### Heart

Heart size can be checked by palpation of the apex, possibly augmented by chest X-ray and/or electrocardiography. Evidence of heart failure can be assessed by listening to the chest and looking for raised jugulovenous pressure.

### Kidneys

Renal function can be assessed by measuring urea, electrolyte and creatinine concentrations in the blood.

### Blood vessels

Check the fundi for retinopathy. The presence of haemorrhages and exudates is a more reliable way of detecting accelerated hypertension than just the presence of papilloedema.

## How can overall risk be measured?

The results of the British Regional Heart Study have suggested a method of quantifying overall CHD risk for an individual patient.[18] Only around half of the variations seen can be explained by the known risk factors, but it is possible to identify a high-risk cohort for especial intervention.

Each risk factor, if present, increases the overall risk between two- and fivefold over those without the factor, so that all factors are of roughly equal importance. The figures apply to men aged 40–60, but it is probably reasonable to extrapolate to other groups.

### Smoking

The number of years for which the patient has smoked at least one cigarette per day          Multiply by 7.5

### Diagnosed CHD

If a doctor has made a diagnosis of angina or MI in the past          Add 265

### Diabetes

If a diagnosis of diabetes has been made          Add 150

### Possible CHD

If the patient has chest pain when walking uphill or hurrying          Add 150

### Family history

If either parent died from a heart attack          Add 50

### Blood Pressure

Take an average of two readings of SBP          Multiply by 4.5

A score of 1000 or more defines a group who have a 10% chance of a major CHD event within 5 years as far as males aged 40–60 are concerned. Corresponding figures for other ages/sexes are:

Men 30–39 – score over 800
Men over 60 – score over 1200
Women over 50 – score over 1200

## 'Will treatment do me any good?'

You will by this stage be able to estimate whether an individual will benefit in a purely medical sense from treatment of the blood pressure. For individuals where mild hypertension is the only problem, the management of the pressure should be the subject of discussion between doctor and patient. The lifestyle constraints, prescription costs and possible side-effects of treatment may be more than the patient is prepared to put up with for such low possible benefits.

The whole point of treating raised BP is to prevent vascular events. For sustained SDP over 200 mmHg and/or sustained DBP over 110 mmHg, the benefits of treatment are considerable.

For lower levels of DBP, the benefits are less impressive. The results of the Medical Research Council trial of mild hypertension suggested that it would be necessary to treat 850 patients with mild hypertension for a year to prevent one stroke.[17] A number of patients would have a stroke in spite of being on medication. It has been estimated[19] that, of 100 patients treated for mild hypertension, 1 will be protected from a morbid event, 6 will experience such an event despite being treated, 10 will suffer side-effects from treatment and all 100 will be 'patients'.

If treatment is being considered, an overall assessment should be made of the patient's cardiovascular risk. Individuals at highest risk have more to gain from treatment of their blood pressure.

If the patient is fully informed about the advantages and disadvantages of treatment of their individual case, many will decline treatment. In many cases the GP will be quite sympathetic to this decision. When a patient does decline treatment, or declines some types of treatment, follow-up is still required as a number of patients will with time progress from the mild to moderate category of risk when treatment is likely to confer more substantial benefits.

## What initial assessment should be made?

When it is agreed that treatment of the BP is to proceed, two questions remain:

- Is there evidence of further end-organ damage not so far found? Referral may be needed.
- Is there a chance that this may be one of the 10% of cases which turn out to be secondary hypertension?

The following assessment is suggested:[20]

## Examination

1. Eyes for arcus and xanthelasma, which may indicate hyperlipi-daemia. Fundi for arterial changes.
2. Pulse for rate and rhythm.
3. Heart sounds for valvular lesions.
4. Heart size for left ventricular hypertrophy.
5. Lungs for left ventricular failure.
6. Abdomen for renal artery bruits.
7. Femoral arteries for coarctation of aorta.

## Investigations

1. Urea and electrolytes, creatinine for renal disease.
2. Urine for protein for renal damage, and glucose for diabetes.
3. Lipids to help in the assessment of overall CHD risk.
4. Electrocardiogram for ischaemia and left ventricular hyper-trophy.
5. Full blood count. Raised haemoglobin is a risk factor for CVA.[15]
6. Chest X-ray in patients over 60. Cardiomegally, aortic aneurysm and evidence of left ventricular fibrillation may be found.
7. Blood glucose for unexpected diabetes.

# How should you treat raised blood pressure?

### Non-drug treatment

This advice should be given to all patients with proven hyperten-sion, and also those awaiting confirmation of diagnosis. An average BP reduction of 10.6/8.1 mmHg may be achieved.[21]

*Smoking*
Smoking should be counselled against.

*Weight control*
Fifty per cent of overweight hypertensives are likely to benefit.[22] Try and get the Body Mass Index below 30.

*Salt*

Opinions vary about the impact of salt reduction, but it seems prudent to advocate a 'no added salt' diet. Potassium chloride is now widely available and is a palatable alternative, without raising the BP.

*Alcohol*

Up to 10% of hypertension is due to excess alcohol.[4] The normal limits of 21 units a week for a man and 14 for a woman apply. Total abstinence is not recommended, as this is associated with increased CHD.

*Exercise*

Exercise helps with diets, lipid levels and generally reducing cardiovascular risk. Thirty minutes three times a week of jogging, swimming or similar is advised. In the sedentary or elderly, brisk walking is recommended.[15] Early surveys suggested the need for exercise to be vigorous before CHD benefits were achieved. Further review of the evidence has emphasized the merit of these lesser degrees of exertion.[23]

*Diet*

A diet to reduce calories and saturated fat ingestion is recommended.

## Drug treatment

Drug treatment should be considered in patients who have not responded to non-drug treatment, and should only be used in conjunction with non-drug treatment.

Reductions in BP of 18.2/12.8 mmHg may be expected from drug treatment.[15] It does not seem to matter much what sort of drug is used – it is the reduction in BP which secures the benefits.

Levels of side-effects are high, especially for the older drugs. For instance, up to 53% of men on hypotensive treatment have some degree of sexual dysfunction, compared with 7% of controls and 20% of untreated hypertensives.[24] Having explained the benefits and drawbacks of drug treatment, it is not unusual for patients to decline medication.

In moderate or severe hypertension – that is DBP over 110 mmHg – drugs can be added in a stepwise manner until control is achieved. After this, the regime can be stepped down again while BP control is satisfactory.

For milder hypertension, drugs should be used separately, and combinations should only be used if control is not achieved. Fifty per cent of hypertensives on drugs will need more than one medicine to achieve control.[15] If a small dose hasn't worked, then it's worth trying a bigger dose. Side-effects can often be avoided by using less than maximum doses of two drugs.

Thiazides or $\beta$-blockers remain the first-line drugs, but newer agents may be first-line if there are problems with side-effects, or other clinical conditions impose restrictions.[25] In a diabetic, for instance, the side-effects of first-line treatments may prohibit their use, and as it seems possible that angiotensin-converting enzyme (ACE) inhibitors may be of benefit to renal functioning, these may be considered first in treating the blood pressure.

*First choice*
*Thiazide diuretics*   remain the first-line drugs at all ages. Smaller doses are just as hypotensive as larger doses but the side-effects are fewer. Potassium supplements are rarely required, but it is prudent to check the urea and electrolyte levels about 4 weeks after the initiation of treatment. If the potassium is below normal, then the addition of a potassium-sparing diuretic such as amiloride 5 mg/day is more effective than using potassium supplements.

Thiazides may aggravate other electrolyte disorders, and should be used with caution in diabetes and avoided in gout. Thiazides may elevate serum cholesterol levels, but there is no proof that this leads to excess CHD morbidity.

In the elderly, thiazides seem to be particularly beneficial.

Bendrofluazide in a dose of 2.5 mg each morning may be used: a dose of 1.25 mg is probably as effective, but there is no tablet of this strength currently available. In some patients bendrofluazide will bring on an unacceptably brisk diuresis, and in this case a longer-acting preparation such as chlorthalidone 50 mg a day can be used.

*Second choice*
$\beta$-Blockers are an alternative first-line treatment. They may be added to a thiazide, or may be substituted if the thiazide has not worked in mild hypertension. Their mode of action in hypertension is unclear. There is a flat dose–response curve, so that if a small dose doesn't work, a larger dose probably won't either, but the chance of side-effects goes up.[20]

Side-effects may be minimized by choice of agent. Atenolol 50 mg daily is probably the $\beta$-blocker of choice. All $\beta$-blockers may precipitate acute asthma, and so should be avoided in the known asthmatic or the patient with chronic obstructive airways disease. They should not be used concurrently with verapamil.

Problems with cold extremities and fatigue may improve if an agent with intrinsic sympathomimetic activity such as oxprenolol is used. Disturbed sleep is less likely with the water-soluble agents such as atenolol.

### Third choice

If thiazides and $\beta$-blockers are insufficient, or if clinical considerations preclude their use, then a third-line agent can be added or substituted.

*Calcium channel blockers*    Calcium channel blockers are roughly as effective as thiazides and $\beta$-blockers but they have not been around as long, so their longer-term safety is less secure. They slow the heart rate and reduce vascular tone. Heart failure may be precipitated, so the utmost care should be used if the patient is already on $\beta$-blockers, and verapamil should not be used at all. Throbbing headache, flushes and ankle oedema may complicate the issue in up to 20% of patients.

Verapamil 240–480 mg/day in two or three divided doses can be used. An alternative is diltiazem in its long-acting formulations at a dose of 120 mg twice a day.

*ACE inhibitors*    ACE inhibitors do not seem to have the same deleterious effect on well-being which is a feature of other treatments for hypertension. In all, 10–25% of patients are troubled by a dry cough. The only major problem in normal use is sudden hypotension, which may occur after the first dose, particularly in patients with renal problems, and in those with heart failure who are taking large doses of diuretics.

ACE inhibitors have potentially hazardous interactions with non-steroidal anti-inflammatory drugs, lithium and potassium salts.

Captopril 12.5 mg twice a day or enalapril 5 mg/day can be used if a diuretic is not being prescribed, but these starting doses should be halved if a diuretic is also being taken. The maximum doses are 150 and 40 mg a day respectively.

*Other agents*    Other agents such as vasodilators, $\alpha$-blockers and centrally acting drugs have now largely been superseded. In difficult cases they are available for use, but side-effects can be considerable.

## What BP level should be aimed for? the J-shaped curve

There seems to be an optimum DBP below which the chance of a CVA or CHD event increases: 80–90 mmHg seems ideal. Treatment of raised BP should therefore aim to get the BP down to 160/90 mmHg.[15] If the treated DBP is under 80 mmHg, then treatment may be reduced, since there is some evidence that excessive lowering of DBP may lead to ischaemic events in the predisposed.

## How long should treatment continue?

In a number of trials of hypertension some patients have managed to stop their medication without obvious ill effect. However, the issue is clouded as the initial diagnosis of hypertension may be in doubt and BP may take a year to start rising after the drugs are stopped. In some of the trials non-treatment groups were given general advice about exercise, weight, smoking, etc.

From a review of the evidence, it may be concluded that medication may be withdrawn in those who are well-controlled, but that long-term follow-up needs to be secured. This stance is supported by the British Hypertension Society.[15] Suddenly stopping β-blockers may unmask angina.

## What follow-up should be done?

Once BP has been brought under control, the patient can be seen less frequently. A monitoring programme should aim to establish:

1. Is the BP well-controlled?
2. Is the patient content with any medication, or have unacceptable side-effects occurred?
3. Is there evidence of end-organ damage which might encourage further lowering of the BP?
4. Are the lifestyle recommendations being adhered to?

If a protocol is available, then a nurse-run clinic is an appropriate place for follow-up of most hypertensive patients. The protocol is more likely to be followed than if the GP is entrusted with it.

At intervals of 3 months the BP should be checked, and rechecked if not satisfactory, and symptoms enquired about.

At intervals of a year the GP can assess progress and results, and make a decision about the need for any further investigations or treatment changes. This depends on the severity of the hypertension, and the compliance of the patient.

## Which patients will benefit from referral?

Referral to a hospital colleague may be considered if:[15]

1. Accelerated or malignant hypertension is diagnosed. An admission is usually needed.
2. The patient is known or suspected to have secondary hypertension. In around 10% of hypertensives the hypertension is a result of another disease process, for instance renal disease. Some of these causes can be cured, and in other instances the hypertension may be worsening the underlying disease process. For both these reasons specialist advice is required.

   Secondary hypertension tends to be more severe and occur at an earlier age than essential hypertension. The nocturnal dip in BP is often absent. Treatment to lower the BP is often ineffective or only partially effective. Unexpected findings when the initial work-up of the new hypertensive is done may give a clue to an underlying cause.
3. There is refractory hypertension which has not been brought under control with two drugs.
4. The patient is aged under 35 years.
5. The BP shows wide fluctuations.
6. Multiple cardiovascular risk factors are present.

## References

1. *Coronary Heart Disease Statistics.* London: British Heart Foundation. 1994
2. Dennis M and Warlow C. Strategy for stroke. *Br Med J* 1991; **303**: 636–8
3. Ryan D. Hypertension: action plan. *Update* 1992; **45**: 799–800
4. Practical aspects of blood pressure management. *Drug Ther Bull* 1991; **29**: 14. (commissioned and researched by the Association of Consumer Research Eds Herscheimer A & Collier J ) pp 53–6
5. Department of Health. *The Health of the Nation.* London: HMSO. 1992
6. Shaper G. Managing hypertension in general practice. *Monitor Weekly* 1994; 51–4
7. Aylett MJ. Control of blood pressure in patients with hypertension. *Update* 1994; **7**: 230–9
8. Hypertension: the facts. *GP* 1989
9. Petrie JC, O'Brien ET, Littler WA *et al.* for the British Hypertension Society. Recommendations on blood pressure measurement. *Br Med J* 1986; **293**: 611–15
10. Conroy RM, O'Brien E, O'Malley K *et al.* Measurement error in the Hawksley random zero sphygmomanometer: what damage has been done and what can we learn? *Br Med J* 1993; **306**: 319–22
11. MacConnell TJ. Ambulatory blood pressure monitoring. *Update* 1993; 11–12
12. Pickering TG, James GD, Boddie C *et al.* How common is white coat hypertension? *JAMA* 1988; **259**: 255–8

13. Wilson JMJ & Jungner G. Principles and practice of screening for disease. *WHO Public Health Paper.* 1968, Geneva: World Health Organization, 34
14. de Swiet M, Dillon MJ, Littler W *et al.* for the British Hypertension Society. Measurement of blood pressure in children. *Br Med J* 1989; **299**: 497
15. Sever P, Beevers G, Bulpitt C *et al.* Management guidelines in essential hypertension. Report of the second working party of the British Hypertension Society. *Br Med J* 1993; **306**: 983–7
16. British Hypertension Society. Treating mild hypertension. *Br Med J* 1989; **298**: 694–8
17. Medical Research Council Working Party. MRC trial of treatment of mild hypertension: principal results. *Br Med J* 1985; **291**: 97–104
18. Shaper G. GP scoring system assesses patient's risk of CHD. *Monitor Weekly* 1994; **7**: 55–7
19. Pickering T. Ambulatory monitoring and blood pressure variability. London: Science Press. 1990
20. Ryan D. Hypertension: the GP's perspective. Update 1992; **45**: 789–95
21. Essential hypertension – management guidelines. *MeReC Bull* 1993; **4**
22. Croft PR, Brigg D, Smith S *et al.* How useful is weight control in the management of hypertension? *J R Coll Gen Pract* 1986; **36**: 445–8
23. Hardmann AE & Hudson A. Walking for health – a closer look at exercise. *Health Trends* 1989; **21**: 91–4
24. Riley A & Riley E. Antihypertensive drugs and sex. *J Sex Health* 1992; **19**: 31–2
25. *British National Formulary.* No. 27 London: British Medical Association/Royal Pharmaceutical Society of Great Britain. 1994

# 2

# Dyspepsia in general practice

## Aims

The trainee should:

- Be able to select those patients with dyspepsia who need further investigation.
- Have sufficient knowledge of the therapeutic options to treat the majority of patients presenting with dyspepsia.
- Be able to make a positive diagnosis of gastrointestinal motility disorders, and treat accordingly.

## How common is dyspepsia?

Dyspepsia is an ill-defined collection of upper abdominal symptoms, including epigastric discomfort, distension, heartburn and flatulence.[1,2] Over a 6-month period as many as 38% of all adults have some dyspeptic symptoms.[3]

Patients with dyspepsia account for 3–4% of general practice consultations.[1] Some 1.5 million working days a year are lost because of it, and NHS prescriptions for treatment cost over £400m a year (1992).[2]

The prevalence of dyspepsia is not changing, though the incidence of peptic ulcer is declining.[1]

## Is dyspepsia important?

Most causes of dyspepsia are not serious and can be left to run their natural course. For persisting dyspepsia, however, it is important to establish a diagnosis:

- Gastric cancer has a better prognosis if it is diagnosed in its early stages. It is plausible that there is a progression of the disease from the localized cancer to the invasive cancer with the passage of time, but there is no way of proving this, as it would not be ethical to leave a localized cancer to see what would happen.

• Appropriate treatment can relieve a lot of suffering, though in many cases treatment can proceed without a complete diagnosis having been made.

The seriousness of the symptoms is only one of the reasons why patients choose to present themselves to their medical advisers. Patients with more severe and prolonged symptoms are probably more likely to visit their GP because of them, but other concerns and beliefs are more likely to inform their decision.

The patient will have talked to family members and may have heard of someone who had a serious stomach pathology: he or she is more likely to consult if he or she believes there may be something seriously amiss,[4] – the so-called perceived vulnerability. Most patients with dyspepsia treat themselves and never attend the doctor. Even so, only 1% of patients presenting to their GP with dyspepsia will have a gastric or oesophageal neoplasm.[1]

There are a number of causes of dyspepsia. Experienced clinicians can achieve a diagnostic accuracy of around 50%. This can be increased to 75% by the use of structured questionnaires.[1]

Gastroscopy has a sensitivity of over 90% for upper gastro-intestinal cancer, with a complication rate of less than 1%. It is the investigation of choice for upper gastrointestinal pathology, and performs significantly better than barium meal.[1]

## What should I do when a patient presents with dyspepsia?

The site and character of the pain, any radiations or associated symptoms and any aggravating or relieving factors should be sought, but this yields poor diagnostic accuracy. Any recent dietary indiscretions, especially with alcohol, may give an insight into the problem, as may a review of prescribed and other drugs being taken, in particular aspirin and non-steroidal anti-inflammatory drugs (NSAIDS).

Severe or persisting pain, vomiting, anorexia and weight loss point to a more sinister pathological process.

At examination, there is usually some epigastric tenderness, but often little else to indicate what might be going on.

Most dyspeptic patients can safely be treated for 4–6 weeks with antacid before any further investigation is required.[1] A simple antacid with or without a rafting agent can be taken either at a dose of 10 ml four times a day, or whenever the symptoms are present. In patients under 45 years old an $H_2$ antagonist can be used with the antacid.

Cimetidine and ranitidine now have non-ulcer dyspepsia as one of their licensed indications, and famotidine and cimetidine are available from pharmacists for the short-term relief of dyspeptic symptoms.[5]

The theoretical danger of the wider availability of $H_2$ antagonists is that it might delay the diagnosis of a gastric cancer, which has an appalling prognosis unless diagnosed and treated in its very earliest stage.[6] However, there is no evidence that the 6-week delay will lead to an adverse effect on the natural course of or surgical cure rate for gastric or oesophageal cancer,[1] and most patients with dyspepsia do not consult their doctor anyway.

## Which patients should be referred straight away?

Patients whose symptoms suggest a cancer need referral without delay. Other cases will also benefit from urgent attention:

- Dysphagia, anorexia and weight loss are suspicious of a cancer.
- Recent substantial gastrointestinal haemorrhage may indicate a need for surgery.
- Patients taking NSAIDs may have the symptoms of any abdominal pathology masked by the medication. In particular, a perforation can occur without any premonitory signs and symptoms.
- Patients presenting with dyspepsia for the first time over 45 years old, or with a change in the pattern of symptoms after this age. Older patients are more likely to have cancer.

When gastroscopy is needed, it should be performed within 4 weeks of referral to ensure early detection of any cancer. Though desirable, this cannot be achieved in most parts of the country. The growing availability of open-access gastroscopy should reduce delays. Most gastroscopies ordered by GPs are done as a precaution and so the formal advice of a gastroenterologist is not required.

## Which patients should be referred later?

Most benign types of dyspepsia will be relieved by a short course of appropriate treatment. If there is a recurrence of symptoms, or if symptoms persist, then further investigation is indicated to exclude a more serious pathology.[6] Reasons to refer are:

- Emergence of symptoms such as vomiting, weight loss, etc.
- Failure of treatment with antacids plus $H_2$ antagonists.
- Recurrence of symptoms after stopping treatment.
- Patients in high-risk groups, such as those with a history of pernicious anaemia, chronic atrophic gastritis or a partial gastrectomy.

## Gastritis

### How does it present?

Shallow breaches in the gastric defences (mucus and epithelium) or erosions may lead to acute epigastric pain, halitosis, especially in the mornings, and occasionally vomiting.[2] Symptoms are usually transient, and often brought on by dietary and particularly alcoholic indiscretion. Antacids will relieve the symptoms.

Clinically there will be localized epigastric tenderness.

Episodes should not last more than a few days.

### What is the treatment?

Many patients with gastritis will already have taken antacids with some relief. They may attend because symptoms are not controlled, because they are persistent, or because they are concerned and would like to know what is happening.

- Avoid aggravating factors, especially alcohol, spicy foods.
- Use antacids in a regular dosage regime until symptoms have been absent for 2 days.
- Prescribe $H_2$ antagonists if necessary for a 2-week course.
- If the symptoms have been brought on by a dietary indiscretion, it is best to avoid this precipitant.

## Peptic ulcer

### Who gets it and why?

Around 5% of people have an ulcer at some stage of their life. The male to female ratio for duodenal ulcers is 6:1; for gastric ulcers the figure is 2:1. They can present in adolescence, but the peak presentation ages in men are 40–50 for duodenal ulcer (DU), and 50–60 for gastric ulcer (GU). In women peak presentations are 10 years later. DUs have a broad distribution among all social groups, but GU is commoner in the more deprived, possibly reflecting their smoking and drinking habits.[2]

An ulcer occurs when the mucus, epithelium and muscularis mucosa are breached, and acid burns the underlying tissue. It arises because of a mismatch between acid plus pepsin on one hand and epithelial cells plus mucus on the other. DU is thought to be due to too much acid, and GU to be due to deficient defences.[2] In both there is a genetic component, so that members of some families and some population groups are at particular risk (for example, the high incidence of DU in Scotland).

There is also an association between peptic ulcer (PU) and chronic bronchitis, ischaemic heart disease, chronic renal failure and alcoholic cirrhosis.[2]

### How does it present?

The classical presentation is of localized epigastric pain which relates clearly to eating in that it is exacerbated by food or hunger. Pain is typically relieved by antacids (even if briefly), bland foods and acid vomiting, and is worse at night. It is a relapsing and remitting disease with relapses lasting 2–4 weeks, and recurrences occurring about every 3–6 months.

Clinically there is localized epigastric tenderness, and the patient is often able to put the tip of the finger on a precise spot where the pain is worst. If there is evidence of anaemia, weight loss and copious vomiting, then a cancer should be suspected, even though a severe ulcer with pyloric stenosis can also give such symptoms. Urgent investigation is required.

### What can be done?

If left alone, a PU will tend to relapse and remit over a 10–25-year period, then resolve. In 1958 a period of hospital rest and stopping smoking was found to help. Up to 25% ended up having some sort of surgical procedure, which sometimes helped. Surgery is rare these days.

In 1976 the first $H_2$ antagonist was introduced and the treatment of PU altered completely. Surgery is now only usually required in an emergency if, for instance, there is bleeding (which still carries an 18% mortality) or if a perforation has occurred as it will in around 5% of cases.

Simple antacids can heal ulcers and bring symptomatic relief. However, the doses have to be very large, and in some preparations the sodium load can cause problems, especially in the more elderly patients and those with renal disease or heart failure. The large doses can also lead to bowel problems. Magnesium-based preparations tend to be laxative, while the aluminium-based ones are constipating. A number of proprietary preparations are available which contain both aluminium and magnesium compounds, but these are more expensive.

Avoiding cigarettes, hot/spicy food and alcohol also helps. Cigarette smoke blocks the effect of $H_2$ antagonists. Smoking doubles the rate of ulcer relapse.[2]

Ninety-five per cent of ulcers can be healed at 8 weeks with $H_2$ antagonists in full dosage. Omeprazole, the proton pump inhibitor, heals them slightly quicker, but the result at 8 weeks is just the same. In those which fail to heal it is worth either doubling the dose of $H_2$ antagonist or trying omeprazole.[7]

The problem with the longer-term management of PU is the relapses. If treatment is stopped at healing, about 85% of ulcers will recur within a year. If half-dose maintenance is used, the relapse is still around 4% a month. Even if maintenance treatment is indicated, a large proportion of patients will only take the tablets when they have symptoms.

**What is *Helicobacter pylori?***

For some time it has been known that the addition of bismuth compounds to ulcer treatment reduces the rate of relapse. It is now clear that the basis of this action is the effect of bismuth on *Helicobacter pylori*.

*H. pylori* is a small flagellate organism which is endemic, and can be found in 20% of 20 year olds and 50% of 50 year olds. However, it is also found in 90% of patients with DU and 70% of patients with GU.[8] At present the best way of detecting it is by sampling the gastric juices at gastroscopy, but breath tests and tests on saliva are becoming available and it may be possible to use these in general practice.

If *H. pylori* can be eradicated in a patient with DU, the yearly relapse rate falls below 20%. With $H_2$ antagonists and omeprazole costing the NHS around £250m a year in 1992, 2% of prescriptions and 10% of all NHS primary care prescribing costs,[9] this difference has considerable economic as well as clinical significance.

## Who should have *Helicobacter* eradication treatment?

In routine practice, attempts to eradicate *H. pylori* should be limited to patients in whom duodenal ulceration is a management problem. It is recommended[8] that eradication should be considered before or after a standard ulcer-healing course of antisecretory therapy where:

- Maintenance treatment is needed.
- Elective surgery is being considered.
- There has been previous haemorrhage or perforation.

As yet there is no known benefit in eradicating *H. pylori* in patients with non-ulcer dyspepsia, gastric ulceration or non-steroidal-induced ulceration.

## How do you eradicate *H. pylori*?

Triple therapy with 2 weeks of colloidal bismuth 120 mg q.d.s., metronidazole 400 mg t.d.s. and tetracycline 500 mg q.d.s. will eradicate *H. pylori* in 93% of cases.[8] With amoxycillin 500 mg t.d.s. instead of the tetracycline, this falls to 73%.

Unwanted effects such as a metallic taste, nausea, vomiting and diarrhoea occur in 50% of those treated. Also, in 20% of cases the organism is resistant to metronidazole.

Double therapy with omeprazole 20 mg/day and amoxycillin 500 mg thrice daily is better tolerated, but cures only 30–80% of infections.

## Which patients need long-term acid suppression?

*H. pylori* eradication treatment is as yet not completely effective. In addition, even if the organism is eradicated, then ulcer relapses can still occur. There may be reinfection. In a number of cases, therefore, symptoms will persist, and in these cases the longer-term use of an antacid, an $H_2$ blocker or a proton pump inhibitor will be required.

Patients in whom long-term acid suppression is indicated are:

- Symptoms under good control.
- Gastric ulcer present.
- Duodenal ulcer present, and symptoms not eradicated by anti-*H. pylori* treatment.
- Gastro-oesophageal reflux disease present (see later).

## Gastrointestinal tract movement disorder: dysmotility

### What is it?

Irritable bowel syndrome (IBS) can affect any part of the gut from the mouth to the anus.[10] Where it appears in the differential diagnosis of dyspepsia the stomach and oesophagus are primarily affected, but there is often evidence of disorder elsewhere as well. In addition the bile duct may be involved,[10] producing symptoms very like gallbladder disease.

Symptoms of glubus, flatulent dyspepsia and recurrent vomiting may be seen.

The cause of IBS can only be speculated at but uncoordinated muscle activity heads the list of theories. IBS symptoms can be reproduced by inflating balloons inside the gut,[11] so that pressure must be a factor. An alternative explanation is that IBS is a psychosomatic manifestation of stress.

### Who gets IBS?

In community surveys about a quarter of adults have symptoms of IBS, of whom about a third consult their doctor.[9] Upper abdominal symptoms are somewhat rarer, and are often found in association with the more characteristic lower abdominal IBS symptoms.

Those who consult for IBS are those with worse pain, abdominal distension, recent adverse life events, higher anxiety and depression scores and a belief that their symptoms indicate a serious pathology. Patients with IBS who do not consult are psychologically indistinguishable from the rest of the population.[12]

Patients with IBS are slightly less sensitive to pain generally than the average, so IBS should not be seen as a generalized hypersensitivity disorder.[13] Sufferers are more likely to have had abdominal pains in childhood, heartburn and general dyspepsia, flushing, palpitations, migraine and urinary symptoms.[11] In one series 70% of the women sufferers had dyspareunia.[14]

### How do you diagnose IBS?

The pain experienced is often variable in severity and site. It is likely to be present in the morning, in contrast to the pain of most organic dyspepsia which comes on as the day proceeds.[10] Despite the pain's reported severity, the patient is usually in robust good health and there is no weight loss or anorexia.

There is often much concern about the implication of the

symptoms. IBS used to be a diagnosis of exclusion, which meant that numerous investigations had to be done to exclude everything else. In patients who are already anxious about their symptoms, the tests and the wait for the results are hard to bear. If a positive diagnosis can be made at an early stage, much worrying and expensive interference can be avoided.

Where there are associated lower gut symptoms, Manning's criteria for IBS can be used.[15] Three or more of the following features should have been present for 6 months to establish the diagnosis:

- Pain relieved by defecation.
- Pain onset associated with more frequent stools.
- Looser stools with pain onset.
- Abdominal distension.
- Mucus in the stool.
- A feeling of incomplete evacuation after defecation.

**Can IBS be treated?**

IBS sufferers should be taken seriously, and their beliefs and concerns discussed. The pains are real. The symptoms could be associated with important abdominal disease. Taking time to explore the patient's agenda is particularly important.

A placebo effect of up to 70% is found for IBS treatments.[13] Pain can be treated with a tricyclic antidepressant in normal antidepressant dosage,[13] though opinion on the effectiveness of this varies.[11] Metoclopramide or domperidone in a dose of 10 mg thrice daily can relieve nausea. Antispasmodics such as mebeverine 135 mg thrice a day or dicyclomine 10 mg thrice a day can help. Peppermint compounds, including peppermint water BP, can ease the flatulence.

The diet should contain adequate amounts of fibre and fluid. Some patients find that particular foods aggravate the symptoms and these should be avoided. Relaxation and hypnotherapy can be useful adjuncts to treatment.

IBS tends to start in early adult life. Seventy per cent of sufferers are free of symptoms after 5 years,[11] however they are treated.

# Gastro-oesophageal reflux disease (GORD)

### How common is GORD?

GORD is four times commoner than PU, affecting around 8% of

the UK population. The commonest age is 60–70 years. Obesity, pregnancy and various lifestyle factors contribute to its presence.[9]

## How does GORD present?

The usual presenting symptom is heartburn, a burning discomfort or pain felt behind the sternum, often appearing to arise from the epigastrium towards or into the throat, and sometimes radiating to the back. Occasionally pain is only felt in the throat.

In addition, there may be regurgitation of bitter gastric contents into the mouth and odynophagia (pain on swallowing). Occasionally there may be cough with possible wheeze and dyspnoea caused by aspiration of gastric contents, or occult anaemia.

Symptoms typically occur within 30 minutes of eating a meal. Bending or lying down may provoke an attack. A large meal, particularly if it contains fat, chocolate, coffee or alcohol may also bring on an episode.

## What causes GORD?

The simplest model for the cause of GORD is that gastric contents get into the lower oesophagus and burn it. The reason for this is that the lower oesophageal sphincter (LOS) fails in its job of keeping the acid in the stomach. Reflux of gastric contents occurs in everybody, but in GORD these juices are in contact with the oesophageal mucosa long enough to cause symptoms.

However, at testing only 50% of GORD sufferers show low LOS pressure. On gastroscopy, about 30% of patients with GORD show no evidence of oesophagitis, and only 60% of patients with demonstrable oesophagitis have symptoms of GORD.[16]

Various foods and drugs may transiently reduce the LOS pressure. Delayed gastric emptying, increased gastric acid production and increased intragastric pressure also contribute. Treatment can be directed at all these areas.

## Who needs investigation?

Investigation is rarely needed, but the investigation of choice is gastroscopy. It is reasonable to try a trial of treatment in most patients with GORD.[9] Investigation is reserved for those who fail to respond, or who show features which might be associated with a more serious disorder.

Persisting oesophagitis may lead to the formation of ectopic gastric mucosa in the oesophagus – a Barrett's oesophagus. This is a premalignant condition. Genuine dysphagia is a particularly worrying symptom and requires early investigation.

It is not uncommon to find evidence of a hiatus hernia on gastroscopy. Current feeling is that this is the effect and not the cause of GORD, as spasm in the oesophagus pulls part of the stomach up into the thoracic cavity.[16]

## What can be done?

*Avoid irritants*
Foods which cause a reduction in LOS pressure are:

● Fats.
● Chocolate.
● Mints.
● Caffeine.

Conversely, protein-rich foods increase LOS pressure.
Drugs which cause reduction in LOS pressure are:

● Calcium channel blockers.
● Nitrates.
● Theophyllines.
● Nicotine.
● Alcohol.

*Lifestyle modification*
● Lose weight if overweight.
● Eat smaller quantities at meals.
● Avoid lying down after meals.
● Elevate the head of the bed by 15 cm. A brick end is ideal.
● Avoid dietary irritants, e.g. spices, fats.
● Avoid wearing tight-fitting clothes.

*Medication*
Simple antacids can be very beneficial if taken at the right time and in sufficient quantity. Half an hour after each meal and at bedtime is about right. Adding an alginate with its alleged rafting property will help 65% of GORD sufferers.[9] For the non-responders, $H_2$ antagonists or omeprazole can be tried. Omeprazole gives better results, with a 65% relief of symptoms at 4 weeks compared with 35% for $H_2$ antagonists. In general, larger doses have to be used than in ulcer treatment, and treatment often has to be continuous.

Prokinetic drugs such as cisapride, domperidone and metoclopramide can be effective in resistant cases. The stomach is emptied quicker and LOS pressure is increased so that there is less reflux.

With drug treatment, it is reasonable to continue for 6 months and then review. If symptoms have gone, then treatment can be stopped. If a relapse occurs, investigation is required.[9] Lifestyle modifications should continue indefinitely.

*Surgery*
Surgery is needed in only a small minority of cases. It has a success rate of 90%, and a mortality of 1%.[16]

# Gallstones

### How common are gallstones?

Gallstones are very common, being found in 6% of men and 12% of women in middle age. In 65% of cases they cause no symptoms at all, and in only 10% is cholecystectomy needed.

If symptoms have occurred, however, there is an 80–90% chance of recurrence over 10 years, and complications are common, so that recurrence carries a 5% mortality over 10 years.[17] Gallstones only need treating if they cause trouble.

Women suffer twice as often as men. Middle age is the commonest time for gallstones to present. Obesity predisposes to the development of symptoms.

### What symptoms may be caused?

With biliary colic, there is recurrent mild to moderate pain localized in the right upper quadrant of the abdomen, with possible radiation to the back and shoulder tip. A meal, especially a fatty meal, may aggravate the pain. At examination there is localized tenderness to palpation, which may increase as the patient takes a deep breath.

In cholecystitis, the site and character of the pain are the same, but it is more severe and there may be associated pyrexia, vomiting and prostration.

Pain not localized to the right upper quadrant is unlikely to be due to gallstones. Performing upper abdominal ultrasound on patients with atypical histories will lead to a lot of gallstones being found, but they will usually not be responsible for the symptoms.

## Which patients need referral?

An acute attack of cholecystitis usually requires admission. The patient is usually quite unwell, and it will be difficult to control the pain and maintain fluid balance outside a hospital setting. It used to be common practice to treat acute cholecystitis conservatively, and then readmit patients for interval cholecystectomy, the theory being that surgical complications are more likely if the operation site is acutely inflamed. Opinions are changing, as the mortality rate with immediate and interval cholecystectomy is the same,[17] and around 10% of patients do not turn up for their surgery.

Episodic biliary colic needs a more relaxed approach. The investigation of choice is abdominal ultrasound, which can in many places be done by GPs on an open-access basis. It takes a few minutes and is painfree. Stones in the gallbladder can be readily visualized, and the diameter of the biliary tree will give a good idea whether there are stones in the bile duct.

## Surgery

About half of patients treated conservatively for gallstones are likely to have a recurrence of symptoms within 5 years.[18] The only sure way of preventing gallstones returning is to remove the gallbladder. There are three options:

### Open cholecystectomy

This traditional operation takes 45–60 minutes, involves a long subcostal incision, and requires 7–10 days in hospital. Operative mortality is under 1%, and virtually unknown in patients under 70. Twenty per cent of patients have complications, which in half of cases is a wound infection. A convalescence of 2–3 months is needed before return to full functioning.

### Minilaparotomy cholecystectomy

A 5–10 cm midline transverse incision is used, and surgery takes about an hour. Four days in hospital are needed, followed by 3 weeks' convalescence. This is only slightly cheaper than the open approach as, though the hospital stay is reduced, the procedure takes longer.

### Laparoscopic cholecystectomy

This is now available in most centres, and offers potential benefits over conventional surgery. Four or five very small (under 1 cm) incisions are made in the abdominal wall, and surgery takes about

75 minutes. The patient is in hospital for 2 days, and thereafter 2 weeks' convalescence is needed. Cosmetic results are excellent.

Concern has been expressed at complication rates. Two per cent of patients have complications after laparoscopic cholecystectomy,[18] with better results being obtained by more experienced surgeons. In addition, in 4% of patients the operation cannot be done for technical reasons and then an open procedure is needed.

### Can surgery be avoided?

Non-surgical treatments for gallstones are reserved for those unable to tolerate surgery. No method is as effective at removing the stones and preventing recurrence as surgery.

Oral deoxycholic or ursodeoxycholic acid will dissolve stones of pure cholesterol up to 0.5 cm across. Treatment has to continue for 2 years, and 3 months after the stones are dissolved. Recurrence is common, as are side-effects (mainly diarrhoea), and the treatment is relatively expensive.

Extracorporeal lithotripsy shakes the stones into little bits so they will pass along the bile duct. Damage to surrounding organs, mainly the right kidney, is not uncommon, and fragments may not pass along the bile duct, requiring an open procedure to remove them. Recurrence is common, and the procedure is currently going out of routine use.

## Upper gastrointestinal cancer

If a diagnosis of gastric or oesophageal cancer has been made, the patient will normally be admitted to hospital for further investigation, staging of the disease, and the consideration of further treatment. Many will subsequently have a spell at home. Though most hospitals offer very good counselling facilities through trained and experienced oncology counsellors, the patient or relatives may none the less turn to their GP for information and advice.

### Will the patient die?

Oesophageal cancer has a 5% cure rate after treatment, with the median survival time after diagnosis being 10 months.[19]

Gastric cancer has an overall cure rate of 5%. If detected at a very early stage, around 70% can be cured, but only 1% of cancers are detected at this early stage. In 80% of cases the tumour is advanced at diagnosis, and in 40% no treatment at all is possible.[20]

Pancreatic carcinoma carries an overall 5-year survival of 5%.

For all these cancers, the stage at which they are diagnosed has more impact on the eventual survival than the treatment used. Spread beyond the mucosa and into the regional lymph nodes carries a much poorer outlook. For example, oesophageal cancers confined to the mucosa and submucosa will achieve a 5-year survival of up to 80% following surgery.[19]

### Can anything else be done?

Radiotherapy has little to offer in upper gastrointestinal cancer.[19]

Chemotherapy has been shown to offer some advantages, especially with advanced cancers. The outlook for such cancers is so poor that even a modest improvement in prognosis is to be welcomed. It is sometimes possible to shrink a tumour or regress its staging so that surgery is more successful.

By the time the diagnosis is made, it is often true that only palliative care is appropriate. With the exception of pancreatic cancer, pain can usually be kept under control. Bone metastasis is not common, and so bone pain is less troublesome. Wasting can be considerable, so that skin care is a priority.

Nutrition and fluid balance are particular concerns with upper gastrointestinal cancers. Any obstructions, particularly of the oesophagus, can be relieved by the use of a stent.

# References

1. Brown C & Rees WDW. Dyspepsia in general practice. *Br Med J* 1990; **300**: 829–30
2. Jones CTA. Peptic ulcers and dyspepsia. *Update* 1993; **47**: 227–33
3. Bouchier-Hayes T. Gastroenterology. *Horizons* 1993; **7**: 155–6
4. Lydeard S & Jones R. Factors affecting the decision to consult with dyspepsia: comparison of consulters with non-consulters. *J R Coll Gen Pract* 1989; **39**: 495–8
5. *British National Formulary* 27. London: British Medical Association/Royal Pharmaceutical Society of Great Britain. 1994
6. Lloyd M. Early diagnosis of gastrointestinal cancer. *The Practitioner* 1992; **236**: 980–3
7. Langman MJS. Omeprazole. *Br Med J* 1991; **303**: 481–2
8. *Helicobacter pylori* – when and how to treat. *Drug Ther Bull* 1993; **31**: No 4, 13–15
9. Gastro-oesophageal reflux disease. *MeReC Bull* 1993; **4**: 17–20
10. Swarbrick E. Pointers to functional gastrointestinal disease. *Gastroenterol Pract* 1994; **9**: 14–16
11. Fry J. Irritable guts in irritable people. *Update* 1993; **46**: 1051–2
12. Kettell J, Jones R & Lydeard S. Reasons for consulting in irritable bowel

syndrome: symptoms and patient characteristics. *Br J Gen Pract* 1992; **42**: 459–61

13. Kamm M. Irritable bowel syndrome – new developments. *Gastroenterol Pract* 1993; **8**: 6–8
14. Stevens R. Irritable bowel syndrome. *The Practitioner* 1992; **236**: 976–9
15. Manning AP, Thompson WG, Heaton KW et al. Towards a positive diagnosis of the irritable bowel. *Br Med J* 1978; **2**: 653–4
16. Bate C, Calam J, Crean G *et al. GP Pocket Guide to Acid Reflux*. London: Astra. 1993
17. Finlayson N. Cholecystectomy for gall stones. *Br Med J* 1989; **298**: 133–4
18. Managing patients with gall stones. *Drug Ther Bull* 1994; **32**: 33–35
19. Ellis P & Cunningham D. Management of carcinomas of the upper gastrointestinal tract. *Br Med J* 1994; **308**: 834–8
20. Allum WH. Gastric cancer. Allum. *Update* 1993; **47**: 87–93

# 3

# Cancer of the breast

## Aims

The trainee should:

- Be able to make a competent examination of a breast lump.
- Be able to counsel the patient who has contracted cancer of the breast.
- Be aware of the breast cancer prevention programme and be able to participate appropriately in it.

## A few statistics

There are about 26 000 new cases of breast cancer diagnosed in the UK each year, and 16 000 deaths.[1] It is the leading cause of cancer death in women aged 40–50.[2] Comparing this with other important cancers in women, there are each year about 4500 cases and 2200 deaths from cancer of the cervix, 5000 cases and 4300 deaths from cancer of the ovary, and 3750 cases and 1000 deaths from cancer of the uterus.[3]

After 5 years, 62% of breast cancer sufferers are alive, compared with 58% for cancer of the cervix, 28% for cancer of the ovary and 70% for cancer of the uterus.[4] The prognosis for advanced breast cancer has altered little in the last 30 years, but the outlook for sufferers from early breast cancer has improved.[5]

The UK has the highest mortality from breast cancer in the world, accounting for 20% of all new cancers and 20% of cancer deaths.[3] The number of breast cancer sufferers is rising throughout the world.[2]

## Which women are at risk of breast cancer?

Each woman in the UK has a lifetime risk of 1 in 12 of contracting breast cancer.[1] Some groups of women are at particular risk:[2]

## Age

Breast cancer is rare under age 30, and the incidence roughly doubles with each decade thereafter until the menopause, when the rate of increase slows appreciably.[6]

## Family history

About 5% of breast cancers are due to highly penetrant dominant genes.[7] If a first-degree relative has had breast cancer under age 40, or if there is also a history of other cancers under age 50, then the woman is at particular risk and needs extra supervision.

## Being a woman

Breast cancer is very rare but not unknown in men.

## Late first pregnancy

Women who have a first full-term pregnancy after the age of 35 carry three times the risk of women who are first pregnant below age 20.[7]

## Early menarche

Women who begin menstruating at age 10 have three times the breast cancer risk of those who begin at 15.[7]

## Late menopause

Women whose periods stop at 55 have twice the breast cancer risk of those who stop aged 45.[6]

## Previous breast cancer

# How does breast cancer present

Around 90% of breast cancers are found by the women themselves or their partners.[8]
Clinical features suggesting a malignant lesion are:

## A lump

Around three-quarters present in this way.[9] Hard craggy lumps which are growing and do not alter with the menstrual cycle are particularly suspicious.

## Tethering

A cancerous breast lump may be fixed to the chest wall or to the overlying skin, causing it to pucker. The nipple may have recently become retracted.

## Axillary mass

Malignant regional lymph nodes are hard and matted, and may be fixed to underlying structures.

## Other features

More rarely there may be swelling of the breast, pain, nipple discharge or Paget's disease of the nipple.

# What should you do when a woman presents with a breast lump?

## History

Relevant questions would include:

- How long has the lump been present?
- Is it changing? Is it growing?
- Does it alter with the menstrual cycle?
- Are there any associated symptoms?
- Is there any personal or family history which might be relevant?

## Examination

It is most important to be able to perform an adequate clinical examination of the breasts. There are a number of ways to examine breasts. Whichever is chosen, it is important to be consistent and careful.

1. Ask the woman to undress to the waist while sitting upright with the arms down. Observe the breast contours.
2. Ask the woman to lift her arms above her head, and observe again.
3. Ask the woman to lie down on a couch with her head inclined at 30°, arms by her sides.
4. Start by examining the asymptomatic breast.

5. Using the flat of the hand or straight fingers, palpate the breast against the chest wall. Either start at the nipple and work outwards in a spiral, or palpate the four quadrants in turn.
6. Feel for axillary lumps.
7. Ask the woman to sit leaning slightly forwards, and palpate the breasts again.

## What can you say to a woman with a breast lump?

Breast pathology is very common, and women are rightly concerned if a lump is found. Only a minority of lumps will turn out to be malignant. If a lump is found which has none of the characteristics of malignancy, then it is reasonable to leave it until after the next period and then re-examine it. Many lumps will disappear after the period, and the woman can be reassured that all is well. If the lump persists, then referral is mandatory. Any new lump found in the breast of a postmenopausal woman requires referral.

A more complete diagnosis of a breast lump can only be made having gone through the triple assessment at a specialist centre.[2]

1. Clinical examination.
2. Fine-needle aspiration cytology (FNAC).
3. Diagnostic mammography.

The clinical examination will be broadly a repeat of the examination already performed, but done by a doctor with a special interest and expertise with breast lumps.

FNAC involves the insertion of a needle, usually of 'green barrel' gauge, into the lump, sometimes under mammographic guidance. This will determine whether the lump is solid or not, and may yield fluid for histological analysis. An anaesthetic is not usually required. Some specialists are so confident in their technique that unless the fluid is blood-stained it is not sent for cytological analysis, and if any cyst can be aspirated to extinction then the woman is discharged from further follow-up.[2]

Diagnostic mammography involves a number of views, and in this respect is unlike screening mammography. In other respects it is similar in that the same equipment is used, and discomfort is relatively minor.[10] About 18% of palpable breast cancers will yield a normal mammogram,[2] and so it is important that this is not the only basis of the diagnosis and that a full assessment is made.

If a decision is made that a breast lump is possibly cancerous, then the patient should be seen by a specialist without delay, within 1 week of referral. Delays may possibly worsen the eventual prognosis, and they certainly increase the psychological burden on the woman.

Units with an interest in breast cancer generally achieve better results from treatment, a topic which has recently stimulated the Cancer Relief Macmillan Fund to campaign for minimum standards to be applied to units treating breast cancer.[11] Such a unit should be available within reach of all patients in the UK.

## 'Am I going to die, Doctor?'

The mortality from breast cancer is related to the stage of the disease.[12]

### Stage I

This stage is a localized lump with no nodes involved. The 5-year survival is 90%.

By further histological typing of the cancer, it is possible to select out a subgroup of very mild cancers (around 11%) whose death rate is the same as the general population.[2]

### Stage II

This stage is a localized lump with nodes involved. The 5-year survival is 60%.

### Stage III

This stage involves locally advanced disease. The 5-year survival is 40%.

### Stage IV

As well as a lump, distant metastases are present. The 5-year survival is 10%. Early breast cancer, the group in which there has been some demonstrable improvement in prognosis, is that in which the tumour is technically resectable.[12] This takes into account a tumour size of under 4 cm across, the absence of palpable axillary nodes, and the absence of extension of the tumour or metastases to the skin or chest wall. In fact, around 50% of breast cancers in which at first no lymph nodes are palpable will by their clinical course confirm that distant metastases must have been present at the time of diagnosis.[2] However, this does not materially affect management.

Eighty per cent of breast cancers present at this early stage.[12]

## What will surgery consist of?

For early breast cancer, mastectomy and conservation surgery with radiotherapy carry an equal chance of survival.[5] Mastectomy is a bigger and more mutilating operation.

Conservation surgery consists either of removing the lump with a tumour-free margin (the so-called lumpectomy), or else removing the breast quadrant containing the tumour. Both these are combined with either axillary clearance or sampling, depending on the views of the surgeon. There is controversy surrounding this issue. Arguments include the following:

### Axillary clearance

• Gives histological evidence for tumour staging.
• Prevents axillary recurrence.

### Axillary sampling

• Gives histological evidence for staging.
• Positive nodes can receive radiotherapy so that the outcome is just as good as with clearance.
• Surgery is less extensive.

Not all tumours can be treated with conservation surgery. Those over 4 cm usually require a mastectomy. However, it is sometimes possible to shrink a tumour down to 4 cm using chemotherapy so that breast conservation can be achieved.[12]

Local tumour recurrence is greater after conservation surgery, at between 5 and 21%.[2] This does not, however, affect the death rate from the disease. It is straightforward to perform a mastectomy after initial conservation surgery.

The psychological consequences of mastectomy and conservation are about the same, with 35–40% of women suffering anxiety, depression or both in the 2 years following each procedure.[5] Though the preservation of the breast has important benefits in terms of self-image, it often means that women are less secure in the belief that the cancer has gone, leading to obsessive concern over breast symptoms.

The best way to secure psychological health after breast cancer surgery is to involve the woman fully in management decisions. There is some evidence that this is being achieved to a greater extent than in the past.[11] This does mean, however, that it is impossible to involve breast cancer sufferers in the randomized trials necessary to improve future treatments.

The cosmetic results after mastectomy tend to improve with time, whereas after conservation surgery the opposite is often the case because of the longer-term effects of radiotherapy.[2]

Breast reconstruction is done in about 10% of women after mastectomy,[13] whereas about 50% would like it. Any problems following the surgery will depend on the particular technique used. Reconstruction does not, however, lead to an increased chance of tumour recurrence.[13]

# Will further treatment be needed?

### Radiotherapy

In women treated with lumpectomy and axillary node dissection, recurrence rates are less if subsequent radiotherapy is used.[5] Treatment is to the tumour bed in all cases, and also to the axilla if the nodes have been sampled rather than cleared. Radiotherapy and axillary clearance together is avoided as this invariably leads to lymphoedema of the arm.

Around 30 treatments are needed over several weeks or months. This will involve repeated visits to the treatment centre. Other problems are that the cosmetic result of surgery tends to be worse because of radiation scarring, and there is an increased incidence of ischaemic heart disease.[2] Larger more focused doses of radiation can be achieved by implants.

### Chemotherapy

Chemotherapy improves the outlook particularly in advanced breast cancer.[1] Death from the disease is not avoided, but life can be prolonged.

In early breast cancer, chemotherapy improves survival by 16% and recurrence by 28%,[5] with benefit being greatest for women under 50 years. However, recurrence and survival rate in this group of patients are very good anyway, so such improvement does not represent much in terms of women alive who would otherwise be dead.

The benefits of chemotherapy have to be balanced against disadvantages. Six treatments are usually needed.[5] The commonest side-effects of treatment are tiredness, nausea, loss of appetite, mouth soreness, pain, sickness and sore eyes. Each patient will have between five and seven side-effects.[14]

## Endocrine therapy

### Ovarian ablation

Ovarian ablation in the under-50 age group reduces recurrence by 26% and improves survival by 25% in early breast cancer.[5] There is an additive effect with chemotherapy.

### Tamoxifen

Tamoxifen is primarily an antioestrogen, but in some respects has oestrogenic properties. Its use improves survival by 17% and recurrence by 25%.[5] It also reduces the chance of recurrence in the other breast by 39%.

Women over 50 do better with tamoxifen, as do those with oestrogen receptor-positive tumours. However, some benefit is seen in all tumour types.

Treatment is known to be effective up to 2 years, and benefits may be seen up to 5 years.

Treatment is usually well-tolerated, though hot flushes, vaginal bleeding and gastrointestinal symptoms can be caused. Its oestrogen agonist properties prevent tamoxifen causing osteoporosis and ischaemic heart disease.

## Psychological support

Most units now have trained counsellors or mastectomy nurses who have often had breast cancer treatment themselves. Early involvement is useful to discuss the nature and implications of treatments.

After or during treatment, a loss reaction is apparent. The female breast serves a wide variety of social and sexual functions. Later, advice about implants and clothing may be useful.

Further support and information can be obtained from self-help organizations:

Breast Care and Mastectomy Association of Great Britain
15–19 Britten Street
London SW3 3TZ
Tel: 0171 867 1103.

British Association of Cancer United Patients (BACUP)
Freeline 0800 181 199 or Information Line 0171 613 2121.

# Can breast cancer be prevented?

The *Health of the Nation* target is to reduce the death rate for breast cancer in the population invited for screening by at least 25% by the year 2000 (from 95.1 per 100 000 population to no more than 71.3 per 100 000).[15]

## Mammography

Screening mammography is a low-intensity X-ray technique which can detect cancers 1 cm or less across. It is slightly uncomfortable, but not unacceptably so.[10]

Surveys during the 1980s confirmed the effectiveness of mammography as a screening procedure to reduce mortality from breast cancer. A 20–30% reduction in mortality can be expected,[16] but benefit is only seen in the over-50 age group. The national scheme started in 1990 for the age group 50–64 years, with repeats thereafter at the request of the woman.

In 1986 the Forrest Report advised the introduction of a national mammography programme in the UK.[22] Only one study, the Swedish two counties study, showed benefit from a 3-yearly single mammogram without clinical examination, but this was the method advised. Other studies which showed benefit in terms of mortality included more views, shorter intervals between tests, or the presence of a clinical examination.

The Forrest Report set targets for the scheme which after the year to April 1992 had all been achieved.[17] Of invited women, 71.3% attended, but this masks large variations between around 50% in inner-city areas, and over 90% in the leafy suburbs.[6] Of those screened, 6.2% were recalled and under 1% of women screened had a biopsy. A total of 6.2 cancers per 1000 screened were detected, with a benign/malignant biopsy ratio of 0.6 : 1. Twenty-two per cent of detected invasive cancers were less than 10 mm across.

If this performance can be maintained, then a 25–30% reduction in mortality from breast cancer is expected, which will comfortably meet the *Health of the Nation* target.

The effectiveness of the programme is limited, particularly in the early years, by a number of factors:[16]

1. The sensitivity of screening mammography is only around 95%.

2. Lead time bias – in the early stages of the programme, some advanced cancers which have been present for a long time may be found. Mortality from these late cases is a lot higher.
3. Length bias sampling – some cancers are detected which are so slow-growing that they would not cause problems during the lifetime of the patient.

Critics of the scheme concentrate on the false-positives and consequent anxiety caused. It is estimated that, of a normal GP list of 2000, 150 will be eligible for screening, 14 will be recalled for further investigation, 2 will have a biopsy and 1 will have cancer.[18] So, for each cancer, 13 others will be unnecessarily worried.

## How is the GP involved in screening?

### Prior notification lists
Population lists are often far from accurate. In inner-city areas Family Health Services Authority registers can be wrong for up to 65% of patients.[19] Before being called for screening, a prior notification list is sent to the GP for confirmation of names, addresses, NHS numbers, sex and suitability for screening.

### Anxiety
Anxiety produced by positive results, either true or false, will have to be coped with.

### Promote screening
Some women will come and ask what the scheme is about, whether it will hurt and whether it would be a good idea for them. The GP is also notified of non-attenders so that the issue can be discussed.

### Counsel
There is no evidence that applying the present screening to the under-50s does any good. Some women will feel cheated at being excluded. If there are grounds for believing that a particular woman is at increased risk of breast cancer, then she can always be referred for assessment through the normal hospital referral channels.

## Should women be encouraged to examine their own breasts?

It is logical to expect an improvement in breast cancer prognosis in women who regularly examine their own breasts and report any lumps found. Women who practise breast self-examination (BSE) are more likely to find lumps less than 2 cm across and are less likely to have axillary deposits at diagnosis.[8]

In population studies, however, BSE has not been shown to reduce the death rate from breast cancer. The only UK population study to show a benefit came from Nottingham, and was based on a cohort who had been taught by a physician how to examine their breasts.[20]

The government's advice to women now is not that they should do BSE regularly, but that they should be breast-aware, and report any perceived changes to their GP.[21]

# References

1. Jones AL & Smith IE. Medical treatment of breast cancer. *Update* 1993; **47**: 505–12
2. Benson JR, Lau Y, Jatoi I *et al.* Early breast cancer: diagnosis and management. *Update* 1993; **47**: 337–44
3. Austoker J & Sharp D. Breast screening: a subject for debate. *Br J Gen Pract* 1991; **41**: 166–7
4. Austoker J. Cancer prevention: setting the scene. *Br Med J* 1994; **308**: 1415–20
5. Management of early breast cancer. *Drug Ther Bull* 1992; **30**: No 14, 55–56
6. McPherson K, Steel CM & Dixon JM. Breast cancer–epidemiology, risk factors and genetics. ABC of breast diseases. *Br Med J* 1994; **309**: 10036
7. Evans DGR, Fentiman IS, McPherson K *et al.* Familial breast cancer. *BR Med J* 1994; **308;** 183–7
8. Fentiman IS. Recent developments in the surgical treatment of breast cancer. *Maternal Child Health* 1992; **17**: 185–90
9. The Yorkshire Breast Cancer Group. Symptoms and signs of operable breast cancer. *Br J Surg* 1983; **70**: 350–2
10. Rutter DR, Calnan M, Vaile MSB *et al.* Discomfort and pain during mammography: description, prediction and prevention. *Br Med J* 1992; **305**: 443–5
11. Cancer charity boosts patients' expectations. *GP Newspaper* May 20 1994;
12. Rubens RD. Management of early breast cancer. *Br Med J* 1992; **304**: 1361–4
13. O'Donnell M. Reconstructive surgery after mastectomy. *The Practitioner* 1994; **238**: 261–265
14. Tierney AJ, Leonard RCF, Taylor J *et al.* Side effects expected and experienced by women receiving chemotherapy for breast cancer. *Br Med J* 1991; **302**: 272
15. Secretary of State for Health. *Health of the Nation: A Strategy for Health in England.* London: HMSO. 1992
16. Michell MJ. Breast screening. *Update* 1992; **45**: 954–8
17. Chamberlain J, Moss SM, Kirkpatrick AE *et al.* National Health Service breast screening programme results for 1991–2. *Br Med J* 1993; **307**: 353–6
18. Austoker J. Breast cancer screening and the primary care team. *Br Med J* 1990; **300**: 1631–4
19. Bowling A & Jacobson B. Screening: the inadequacy of population registers. *Br Med J* 1989; **298**: 545–6
20. Locker AP, Caseldine J, Mitchell AK *et al.* Results from a seven year programme of breast self examination in 89 010 women. *Br J Cancer* 1989; **60**: 271–5
21. Calman KC & Poole AAB. PL/CMO(91)15. London: Department of Health. 1991
22. Forrest P. Breast Cancer Screening 1986; London: HMSO

# 4

# The management of warts in general practice

## Aims

The trainee should:

- Be able to recognize the common manifestations of wart virus infection.
- Know the natural history of a wart and be able to use this knowledge in discussion with the patient.
- Know of a range of harmless and cheap remedies for warts.

## Who gets warts?

Warts have been around for a long time. Celcus in the first century AD described four types of wart. Galen tells of a man who went around the streets of Rome sucking out and biting off plantar warts.

The infectivity of warts was first described in 1891 by Payne. At the time he was treating warts with compounds of salicylic acid, much as is done today.[1] The human papillomavirus (HPV) was identified in 1950.[2]

Ten per cent of people have at least one wart at some time during their life.[3] In institutions it tends to be higher, with an incidence up to 25%.[4] Warts are more common in children, though the incidence in adults may be underestimated.[5] Both sexes and all social classes are affected.

Some people seem particularly prone to warts. In one study new warts were three times commoner in those who had previously been infected.[4] Some occupational groups are at extra risk, in particular fishmongers, poultry processors and butchers.[3,5]

# What causes warts?

Warts are caused by varieties of the HPV. At the last count, 55 different HPVs had been identified,[6] called HPV1, HPV2 and so on. The commonest types are 1–4, but others are also significant, for instance HPV16 is associated with cervical cancer. Fourteen types are only found in epidermoplasia verruciformis, a congenital condition characterized by multiple warts which frequently undergo malignant change.

HPV is transmitted from person to person, or via fomites. It can survive down to −25°C,[3] and is viable for short periods on warm wet surfaces such as the sides of swimming baths. The virus enters through breaches in the skin. It may lie dormant in skin for months or years.[2] Incubation may take anything from a few weeks up to a year.[6]

The type of wart which develops depends on the site where it occurs, and the type of HPV involved.

# What happens to warts?

If left alone, warts may last for up to 5 years.[2] Twenty per cent will have resolved after 3 months, 30% after 6 months[1] and 50% at 2 years.[3] Warts may regress in different ways, the process usually taking 3–4 weeks. Some silently shrink away, others become swollen and inflamed, and yet others undergo haemorrhagic necrosis.[2]

The resolution of the wart and its response to treatment depend on the type of HPV involved, the quantity of virus present and, most importantly, the immunological status of the patient.[1] Patients with immunological disorders such as leukaemia and Hodgkin's disease and those on immunosuppressive treatments are prone to multiple warts which are resistant to treatment. Even minor immunological disturbances such as atopic eczema can give rise to difficult warts.

It is the immune system which eventually kills the virus and causes resolution of the wart. After cure or spontaneous resolution, antibody levels are maintained for about 4 years and then decay.[1] Immunity to one type of HPV does not give much protection against infection with other types.

# What are the different types of wart

Warts are usually quite easy to diagnose because of their characteristic appearances. If there is doubt, the top of the lesion should be pared down slightly. If it is a wart, this will reveal small black spots which are the ends of thrombosed capillaries – a characteristic histological feature of warts.

### Common wart

This is the typical wart, usually found on the fingers and back of the hands. A mound of keratin develops which causes the characteristic shape. HPV2 is the usual cause.

### Plantar wart or verruca

This is also caused by HPV2. The flattened appearance is thought to be due to compression forcing the wart to grow into the skin rather than outwards. The plantar wart may be painful, especially if it is in a weight-bearing area.

### Filiform wart

The filiform wart grows out like a little bush. The most common site is the face.

### Anogenital wart

These are often multiple and occur in the genital tract. Transmission is usually sexual, and there may be other sexually transmitted diseases present. Occasionally they are seen in children, which may give rise to suspicion of sexual abuse. However the virus can also be transmitted during childbirth from the genital tract of an infected mother.

Genital warts are a risk factor for carcinoma of the cervix. Typically the cause is HPV16, but HPV6, HPV11 and HPV18 also occur.

### Plane wart

These are small, flat and usually multiple. They are commonly found in children, and often on the face. They are not visually very obvious.

### Periungual wart

These are common warts which develop at the nail margins. Children who suck their fingers, causing skin maceration, or those who bite their nails create breaches in the skin to allow entry of the virus. The nail bed may be damaged, resulting in a distorted finger nail. Periungual warts are particularly resistant to treatment.

### Mosaic warts

These are groups of small warts found typically on the soles of the feet or round the nails, and are caused by HPV2. Treatment is very slow and difficult.

### Molluscum contagiosum

This is caused not by an HPV but by a pox virus. Multiple small umbilicated lesions are seen, often on very small children, and commonly on the face. They are not as durable as most warts.

## Are warts worth treating?

The literature on warts is divided fairly evenly between those who advocate treatment,[1] and those who think warts should be left to resolve themselves.[7]
   Arguments for treating warts:

• Warts are unsightly and can be painful.
• Treatment of warts can make them go away more quickly.
• If warts are treated more quickly, the pool of infection in the community is reduced. This protects everyone and in particular those at risk of multiple resistant warts, such as the immuno-suppressed.
• HPV cannot be killed by treatment, it can only be killed by the body's cellular immune system. Treating the wart stimulates the body's cellular immunity.[1]

Arguments against treatment are:

• Warts are not fatal, except in the very rare instances where unusual types of HPV cause possibly pre-malignant lesions in patients with epidermoplasia verruciformis. The presence of HPV on a cervical smear is known to be associated with an increased

chance of the patient developing cervical cancer, but the precise role of the HPV is as yet unclear.[2]
- Warts always eventually resolve themselves.
- Treatments for warts can be messy, tedious and painful, and often do not work.
- Treating patients for warts uses health resources and raises expectations.

## What treatments are available?

### Surgical

*Curettage*
This method is effective, but leaves a scar and recurrence is common.

*Operative*
Historically a number of mutilating procedures have been tried; for instance, in Dickson's procedure the verruca, toe and part of the metatarsal head are removed.

### Cryotherapy

This is usually done with liquid nitrogen at minus 196°C. It can be applied with a cotton bud, or better, with a spray. The 12-week cure rate is 50–80% using an average of two to three up to six applications at 2–4-weekly intervals.[5] Treatment is painful. Success is greatest with common warts on the hands. The addition of a daily application of a wart paint can increase the success rate to near 90%.[8]

A container of liquid nitrogen costs around £500 (1989), which translates to about 50p per application. Unfortunately, the procedure does not attract a minor surgical fee. The nitrogen is applied until a white halo 1 mm wide forms round the wart. It is left to warm, and then repeated at the same visit. The mechanism of action is not fully clear, but the formation of ice crystals and their subsequent melting probably damage the cells.

### Paints and ointments

Most are based on salicylic acid, lactic acid and copper plus or minus collodion. Salicylic acid is a keratolytic and also disrupts cell adhesiveness. Lactic acid works by applying a pH load to the wart. Collodion keeps the chemicals fixed in place without having to use a plaster.

Treatment is applied once a day. The wart is prepared by a 10-minute soak in warm water. The skin is dried, and then any loose skin is gently rubbed off with a pumice or emery board. This rubbing should not be too vigorous or the normal surrounding skin will become inflamed. The mixture is applied carefully to the wart, allowed to dry, and then left until the next day when it needs peeling off before the next treatment.

After 12 weeks' treatment, 70–80% of common warts and verrucae will have gone, but only 40–50% of mosaic plantar warts will have resolved.[5]

## Other treatments

*Intralesional injection*
Interferon or bleomycin can be injected.

*Soaks*
Formalin and glutaraldehyde are used. This is worth trying for resistant plantar warts.

*Podophyllin*
This is particularly useful for anogenital warts. It is teratogenic in pregnancy.

*Hypnosis*
Hypnosis has been shown to accelerate the cure of warts and reduce their recurrence.[8]

*Wart charming*
There is a long folk tradition of treatments for warts. About 12% of patients attending a wart clinic will previously have tried a folk remedy, usually because of a hand wart.[9] There are four categories of remedy:

1. *Wasting.* The wart is rubbed with something which is then discarded. As the item decays, so does the wart.
2. *Transference.* The wart is rubbed with something which is then left for someone else to find. The finder then takes the wart as well.

3. *Incantations.* The individual uses incantations or employs a charmer.

4. *Specifics.* The wart is rubbed with a widow's wedding ring, dandelion milk, holy water, early-morning spit or urine.

## 'Best buy' treatments in general practice

Most warts do not present to the GP. They are either left alone, or the patient self-treats. For those which do present, the desirability of treatment will depend on negotiations between doctor, patient and usually a parent. In some cases confirming the diagnosis and an assurance that the lesion will eventually resolve without leaving any evidence are all that is required.

If treatment is desirable, insisted upon, or both, then the chosen method will depend on what the GP has available. Paints and ointments, with or without plasters or collodion, are available by prescription, or on over-the-counter sale. The availabilty of cryotherapy and curettage are less widespread in general practice, but can be accessed through dermatology clinics.

Whatever the treatment proposed, the patient must be aware of its side-effects and likely limitations as well as benefits. In treating a minor, it is worth confirming that the child wants treatment. It is not justified to cause a child pain because of a self-limiting lesion which is only causing a problem to a parent who does not like the look of it.

Whatever the treatment, patients should be advised to keep the skin round the wart dry to avoid softening of the keratin and consequent spread of the virus. Cotton socks should be worn for verrucae. Nail biting should be discouraged for periungual warts.

### Hand and face warts

Hand and face warts are best treated with cryotherapy or, failing this, keratolytic preparations.

### Foot warts

Foot warts usually respond to keratolytics, though cryotherapy may also help.

It is not necessary to exclude children with warts from swimming baths. Being unable to swim may lead to drowning, whereas verrucae are never fatal. Many children with HPV infection are quite unaware of their infectivity, so that excluding the patient will make little impact on the public health.

Not all teachers and swimming bath attendants share this view. If there are problems, then treatments involving plasters and collodion will create the appearance that the verruca is under cover and so not infectious. The use of verruca socks is effective. Or you could just suggest that the patient is economical with the truth.

### Mosaic plantar warts

Mosaic plantar warts are very resistant to treatment. Plasters of 20 or 40% salicylic acid can be cut to shape and applied to the area. Soaks in 3% formalin solution may work.

### Genital warts

Genital warts are the province of the genitourinary clinic. Treatments are toxic (podophyllin), and there are often other sexually transmitted diseases present which need follow-up.

### Plane warts

Plane warts can often be left alone. If not, 2% salicylic acid cream can be tried.

### Molluscum contagiosum

Molluscum contagiosum can often be left alone to resolve. If not, each lesion can be pricked with a cocktail stick and given a squeeze.

## Which patients will benefit from referral?

Around 25% of all new referrals to dermatology clinics are because of warts.[6] In up to 8% of cases, lesions referred as warts are in fact something else.[9]

Referral is required if:

- Treatment is unsuccessful after 3 months.
- Persistent pain is a problem.
- The patient is at high risk, especially if immunocompromised.
- Anogenital warts are present.
- Warts are multiple.
- There is doubt about diagnosis.
- A treatment is needed which is not available in the practice.

# References

1. Bunney MH. Viral warts and their management. *Dermatol Prac* 1988; 8–16
2. Bunney MH. Viral warts: a new look at an old problem. *Br Med J* 1986; **293**: 1045–6
3. English J. Warts: a common viral condition. *MIMS* 1988; **15**: 42–5
4. Massing AM & Epstein WL. Natural history of warts. *Arch Dermatol* 1963; **87**: 306–7
5. Keefe M. Viral warts. GP med top 100. *GP Newspaper* June 3 1994; 3748
6. Garioch JJ. Viral warts. *Maternal Child Health* 1992; **17**: 260–4
7. Colebrook M. Warts and verrucae. *Update* 1992; **45**: 452–5
8. Steele K. Treatment of cutaneous warts. *R Coll GP Members Reference Book* 1989; 251–4
9. Steele K. Wart charming practices among patients attending wart clinics. *Br J Gen Pract* 1990; **40**: 517–8

# 5

# Back pain

## Aims

The trainee should:

- Be able to assess and treat the patient presenting with acute back pain.
- Have knowledge of the preventive strategies available for back pain.
- Be able to identify the needs of the patient with chronic back pain, and refer appropriately.

## How important is back pain?

In 1988–9, 52.6 million working days were lost in the UK because of illness certified as back pain. This represents 12.5% of all working days lost because of ill health, and is the biggest single cause of lost days. It has been estimated that the consequent loss of production amounts to £2000m.[1]

Time lost because of back pain doubled from 1970 to 1980, and doubled again from 1980 to 1990.[2] The reasons for this are unclear since, in general, jobs are becoming less physically demanding. It may be that when the unfit back is subjected to strain, it is more likely to become painful. Chronic back pain sufferers who have been off work for 2 years or more rarely return to employment.[3]

Back pain is the single biggest cause of chronic sickness for people in the 16–44 age group.[2]

About 90% of all back pain episodes are managed by the patient and not brought to medical attention.[3] GPs manage most cases of back pain which they see without resort to specialist care.

## Acute back pain

In all, 80% of people have an episode of back pain at some time in their lives.[3] Usually the lower lumbar and sacral areas are affected. Leg pain down as far as the knees is not uncommon, and should be distinguished from sciatica where the pain progresses over the outside of the lower leg and into the heel and foot.

Up to 90% of acute back pain has settled by 2 weeks, and in up to 40% of cases no time is lost from work.[4] However, 89% of patients will have a recurrence, and over the course of 10 years 77% will have some time off with their back symptoms.[1] Only about 10% of cases of acute low back pain will have signs of nerve root entrapment.[3]

## What can the GP do for acute back pain?

It is estimated that there are 2 million GP consultations a year because of back pain.[1]

With an acute back pain the GP has two priorities:

1. Rule out any of the serious pathologies which might be causing the pain.
2. Control the pain.

### Excluding serious disease

In only 10–20% of cases can a definitive diagnosis be made.[3] Most back pain falls into the category of mechanical back pain, which is either the result of abnormal stress on normal tissue, or of normal stress on abnormal tissue.[1]

In patients who develop back pain aged under 55, serious pathology is very rare. By the same token, back pain presenting for the first time in a patient over the age of 55 should give rise to concern and a search for an underlying serious disease process such as neoplasia or an osteoporotic collapse.

The differential diagnosis of back pain is extensive and, apart from the largest category of mechanical back pain, includes:[1]

- Degeneration – of discs, joints.
- Inflammation – ankylosing spondylitis (70% of cases present with back pain[2]) or rheumatoid arthritis.
- Infections – osteomyelitis, abscess, tuberculosis.
- Neoplastic – myeloma, lymphoma, cancer (usually secondary, primary sites being lung, prostate, thyroid, kidney, breast).
- Metabolic – osteoporosis, osteomalacia, Paget's disease.
- Other – sickle-cell disease, claudication.

In practice the important thing to exclude in the acutely presenting back is a neurological lesion resulting from the back pathology. In particular, a cauda equina lesion causing loss of sphincter function and anaesthesia in the typical saddle distribution is a surgical emergency.

## Controlling the pain

*Posture*
The posture of least pain should be adopted. Lying down on a firm surface is usually most comfortable. Pillows can be placed under the knees, or between the knees if a side position is more comfortable. In some cases, however, the sitting position will produce the least pain.

The traditional method of treating acute back pain was to put the patient to bed for 3 weeks. It is now known[4] that this is far longer than necessary, and leaves the patient open to stiffness, muscle loss and deep venous thrombosis. Two days' bedrest is sufficient in most cases.

*Medication*
Analgesics should be used, starting with paracetamol 1 g four times a day, and if necessary increasing the potency up to and including opiates. They can be effectively used in conjunction with non-steroidal anti-inflammatory preparations such as ibuprofen up to 1800 mg a day in divided doses.

Muscle spasm is often an important component of the symptoms, in which case a short course of an antispasmodic such as diazepam may be helpful. Bedrest and strong analgesia often lead to constipation, which is best avoided by using a softening laxative such as lactulose.

*Other treatment*
Strategically placed cold or hot packs may relieve spasm and ease pain.

When an acute episode is not settling, the early introduction of physiotherapy may help. In the patient under 55 with an acute disc lesion, the McKenzie regime may be recommended by the physiotherapist. In this, exercises are done which produce progressively more spinal extension. This has the effect of milking the disc back into place.

Of the other physical therapies available, chiropractic has been shown to hasten the improvement in acute back pain.[1]

*Exercises*
As the pain begins to ease, usually after 1-2 days, the next priority

is to make sure the back doesn't get stiff as this will prolong symptoms and disability. If muscles are not used they lose 3% of their strength each day.[5]

1. Start non-weight-bearing exercises.[6] These should be done every 2 hours. They are designed to maintain mobility and to strengthen the abdominal muscles. Up to 40% of the stress going through a back can be taken by the abdominal muscles if they are strong enough.[7]
   The pain should be no worse after the exercises than before.
   - *Pelvic tilt*: Lying on the back, put a hand under the lumbar spine and use the back to press the hand downwards.
   - *Knee rolling*: Lie on the back with the knees bent. Keeping the knees together, rock them from side to side.
   - *Chest to knee*: Still on the back, pull one knee at a time up towards the chest. The hand may be used to help if needed.
2. Start gentle mobilization as soon as the pain permits.
3. Be sure that the lumbar lordosis is being maintained at all times.

## Which patients need admission?

It is rare to have to admit a patient with acute back pain. Hospital care has little to offer that cannot be secured at home. None the less, there are approximately 100 000 admissions a year in the UK for back pain.[4]

Reasons to admit include:

- Pain not controlled.
- The patient is unable to rest adequately because of lack of home support.
- Bowel or bladder signs are present. If acute retention occurs, there may be permanent damage within 12 hours unless the problem is dealt with.

## Which patients need referral?

Each year in the UK 300 000 patients are referred to outpatient clinics because of back pain.[1]

Reasons to refer include:

- No response to treatment after 4 weeks.
- Neurological deficit. These may respond to surgery.

- Diagnosis not clear.
- Access to services which may not be otherwise available, e.g. physiotherapy
- Patient request for a second opinion.

## Making an assessment of the acute back

Even in the acute stage of a new episode of back pain, it may be possible to pick out the cases which are likely not to be in the mechanical category, or which are likely to run a more prolonged course.

### The history[3]

What is the patient's general health like? Has there been an injury? Where is the pain? Where does it radiate? Does anything make it better or worse – coughing, posture, exercise? Any relevant family or occupational history?

What is the pain like? Has the same pain happened before? If so, what has helped it? Is there a question of compensation or litigation?

The features of mechanical back pain are:[1]

*Site*
One or more of:

- Discomfort across lower back.
- Central pain, usually over L5.
- Leg pain or paraesthesiae within the sciatic distribution.
- Unilateral or bilateral buttock or lateral back pain.

*Character*
- Episodic or cyclical pain in the mid-years of life.
- Arises from L3 to S1.
- Early morning stiffness or pain eases when the patient is up and about.
- Relation to posture: often aggravated by sitting or standing still and eased by walking normally. Pain which is greatly worse on walking may indicate either vascular claudication or spinal stenosis.

### The examination

- *Look* at how the patient walks into the room, sits down and gets on to the couch. Is there scoliosis? What is the range of movement of the back?

- *Palpate* the spine to find tender spots.
- *Test* for neurological involvement:
  L4 lesion: Weak quadriceps. Dull sensation over the medial calf.
  L5 lesion: Weak foot eversion. Unable to stand on heels. Weak [dorsiflexion of] big toe. Sensory change outside of shin.
  S1 lesion: Weak plantarflexion. Unable to walk on toes. Reduced power of plantarflexion in the big toe. Sensory change over the achilles tendon.
  Cauda equina lesion: Loss of rectal tone (do a PR (per rectum or digital rectal examination) if suspicious), and sensory changes in the saddle area.
- Other examinations may be suggested from the history and findings. Possibilities include:

  Peripheral vasculature.
  Hip joints.
  Abdominal examination for masses, aneurysms.
  PR for prostatic pathology.
  Skin for psoriasis.
  Hands and thumbs for hypermobility syndrome.
  Weight for obesity.
  Breasts for occult carcinoma.

## What about an X-ray

In most cases an X-ray of the lumbosacral spine does not help with diagnosis. Ninety-five per cent of the over-55s show evidence of degenerative changes in the spine on X-ray,[8] but there is little correlation between X-ray signs of degeneration and the degree of symptoms.

In addition, the radiologists get upset about the work and wasted resources of unnecessary exposure to X-rays. Fifteen per cent of all medical X-ray exposure is because of back X-rays, which may be extrapolated to infer that they cause 19 deaths per year in the UK.[8]

On the other hand, the lumbar spine X-ray, like all investigations, carries powerful magic as far as most patients are concerned. So long as you are fairly sure there is no serious disease process, an abnormal X-ray may help to calm the situation and provides at least a sort of diagnosis.

The Royal College of Radiologists[8] suggests an X-ray:

- If the pain is worsening or not resolving.
- If there is a history of trauma.

• If there is evidence of neurological deficit.

In practical terms an X-ray is probably helpful for pain which is atypical (that is, not mechanical), which has lasted over 4 weeks, or which has arisen for the first time in a patient under 25 (for congenital lesions) or over 55 (for neoplastic lesions).[1]

## Preventing the next attack

In most patients back pain is a recurrent problem. Maintaining general fitness and back mobility can help prevent recurrence. In particular, building up the abdominal muscles will protect the back.

1. Take care with posture when standing, sitting, working and at night in bed. The back should be straight with the shoulders back and the buttocks tucked in. The lumbar lordosis should be retained.
2. Take care when lifting. Does the load have to be lifted at all? Keep a straight back and get as close to the load as possible. Try and bend the knees and so use the legs for the lift.
3. Keep fit. The exercises described above for the relief of acute pain are a good start. Improving general fitness will maintain flexibility and make muscles less likely to tear.

Other good exercises are:

• Lie on the back with the knees bent. Run the hands down the thighs to the knees and so tighten the abdominals.
• On all fours on the floor, flex and extend the lumbar spine repeatedly.
• Lie on the side and curl up, pulling the knees under the chin. Uncurl slowly.

## Chronic back pain

In some cases back pain goes on to run a chronic unremitting course. In an average health district of 250 000, between 50 and 1000 patients will be so disabled.[1] It is generally felt that back pain which has not resolved at 3 months should be seen as a different entity from acute back pain.

In this group, unlike the acute backs, anxiety and depression are overrepresented[9] but whether this is cause or effect is not clear. Eligibility to injury benefit is a better predictor of persisting pain than any other factor, including the severity of the initial pain or the severity of any trauma.[4] Psychological and social issues are at least as important as physical issues.

Other factors predicting a poor outcome include poor posture, repeated lifting, inappropriate leisure activities, poor bed or mattress, poor sleep posture, getting in or out of bed improperly, sitting for longer than 30 minutes (particularly when driving), recurrent bending, stopping preventive exercises, taking no medication, using a corset and general lack of physical fitness.

In addition, pain following trauma can result in two specific syndromes to be tackled.

- Myofascial pain is characterized by multiple areas of local irritability (trigger points).
- Sympathetically maintained pain is where proximal trauma leads to distal burning pains and sympathetic imbalance (changes in temperature, colour and sweating).

## What can be done for chronic back pain?

### Medication

Simple analgesics with or without non-steroidal anti-inflammatory drugs (NSAIDs) can be useful. The response to analgesic combinations such as co-proxamol is frequently disappointing and no better than paracetamol alone.[5] Ibuprofen 400 mg three or four times a day in addition to paracetamol 1 g (two tablets) four times a day are suitable choices.

Stronger narcotic analgesics are addictive and suppress natural endorphin production. They should be avoided in chronic back pain.

Antispasmodics such as the benzodiazepines are similarly unhelpful. Not only are they addictive, but the pain is unlikely to be due to muscle spasm anyway.

Tricyclic antidepressants are sometimes but not always useful. Used in full dosage for instance, 75–150 mg amitryptiline a day) they will often work as a co-drug with analgesics. If there is no response after 6 months they should be discontinued.[3]

### Exercises

Rest tends to be favoured by patients with back pain since pain levels are reduced by relieving the load on the back and not stimulating the pain receptors. When exertion is attempted, the subsequent aching of the deconditioned muscles reinforces the view that exercise makes things worse. Corsets and braces are merely ways of resting a particular part of the back.

Exercise on the other hand has a number of positive benefits, even though more pain is produced in the early stages. Blood supply, articular function and muscle strength are enhanced, so preventing ischaemia, contractures and wasting. There is increased endorphin production which boosts mood and relieves pain and distress. Independence is reinforced and illness behaviour is reduced.

Suitable exercises are aimed at general fitness while preventing back trauma. General exercises would include non-jarring exertion such as swimming or walking for 20 minutes three times a week. Specific back exercises have been described above.

### Other ways of relieving pain

Manipulation has not been shown to help pain in the long term, but can be used to secure temporary relief so that an exercise programme can be started.

Acupuncture has been shown to be useful,[1,3] but is not generally available on the NHS because of continuing concern about the accreditation of practitioners.

Chiropractic is of proven benefit in chronic back pain.[1] It is not generally available on the NHS.

Transcutaneous electrical nerve stimulation is worth a try, although its value is not certain. The physiotherapy team will be experienced in its use and can give advice.

Local injections can be used, but the necessary skills are not universally available among GPs.

### Diet

Fish oil, particularly cod liver oil, and evening primrose oil are widely promoted for the relief of chronic arthritic pain, at least by their manufacturers. The pain and inflammation of back pain is mainly mediated through prostaglandins (PGs) in the $PG_2$ series. The theory is that increasing the dietary intake of fish oil and evening primrose oil will increase the levels of $PG_3$ and $PG_1$ respectively. These are less inflammatory than the $PG_2$ series.

In practice the doses needed to secure such a change are huge and unpalatable. They can also work out expensive as neither is available on prescription for this indication.

On the other hand, attention to diet will ensure adequate intakes of calcium, iron and vitamin D, as well as keeping a check on the weight gain which often accompanies chronic immobility.

## Psychological support

In a proportion of patients all efforts to relieve the pain fail. In these unfortunate patients the emphasis shifts. Efforts must be concentrated on helping them cope despite their pain, while at the same time not neglecting anything which might bring relief.

Most of these patients will already have been referred because of non-response to treatment. None the less, the GP remains pivotal in their treatment as he or she must reinforce the other efforts which are being made, and is also the most accessible professional in case of problems. The specialized pain clinic, as well as having skills in other pain relief techniques, will also concentrate on the psychological aspects of chronic pain. This approach may well seem strange to the patient, and its validity will need to be reinforced by the GP if the full benefits of the treatment are to be secured.

Using a popular model,[5] the chronic pain causes distress. This distress produces illness behaviour which reacts with the outside world. The illness behaviour is self-reinforcing, and so disability results from a combination of the original disorder, the distress and the illness behaviour. Unless each of these is addressed, there will not be a resolution to the problem. Illness behaviour is sometimes referred to as learned helplessness.

There has to be initial agreement that the pain is the property of the patient, and the main responsibility for coping with it is the patient's. The doctor must also accept the presence of the pain. The distress of the patient is real, and even if there are psychological dimensions to its management, this does not mean that the pain is imaginary or being made up by the patient.

The treatment of chronic pain is prolonged and complex, and does not fit in with the ordinary textbook descriptions of pain management. The pain is almost never completely cured. The GP who is unfamiliar with chronic pain management may find this difficult to come to terms with.

Successful chronic pain management will involve a prolonged doctor–patient relationship characterized by disappointing progress followed by setbacks and emotional upset. The GP should settle in for a long and bumpy ride.

The best results are obtained with a multidisciplinary approach. Back schools and pain clinics exist in many areas to employ just such an approach.

*Assessment*

Start at the beginning and try and find out how much of the problem is caused by the physical problem, how much by the distress, and how much by the illness behaviour. Has an identifiable psychiatric disorder (such as depression) occurred which is delaying recovery? Is there any secondary gain in the illness behaviour.[9]

*Explanation*

Using diagrams and models where possible, try and explain exactly what the back problem is. Go on to discuss the behavioural component to the disability.

Chronic pain serves no useful biological function. Most ordinary pain is caused by tissue damage, and so it is reasonable to infer that avoiding pain will also avoid further damage. This is not the situation with chronic pain, and the patient will need encouragement to persevere with activities which may be causing pain. The disincentives to activity are not only the pain itself but also the assumption that more damage is being done.

*Relief of the pain*

All possible efforts should be made to reduce the physical pain.

*Recovery of function*

Targets for improvement can be set. These might include the recovery of normal muscle tone and joint flexibility. Behavioural objectives might be the resumption of self-care and light daily activities. Formal behavioural therapy may be employed to focus the responsibility for the pain and disability on the patient, and to increase the patient's belief in his or her ability to control the pain and improve coping skills.

*Rehabilitation*

There can be an agreed graded return to normal levels of employment, social and leisure activities.

*Prevention*

Weight control, posture, exercises and fitness and ergonomics will all have a bearing on the prevention of recurrence.

Using similar principles, an intensive course in Finland[4] reported 85% success in getting patients back to work.

*Self-help*

A number of advice leaflets and books are available for people with chronic pain. One such[10] suggests ways of getting the best out of the available services:

- Accept the fact of the chronic pain.
- Set specific goals for work, hobbies, social activities.
- Let yourself be angry if the pain is getting the better of you.
- Take analgesics on a strict time regime, then taper off.
- Get fit and stay fit.
- Learn how to relax and practise regularly.
- Keep yourself busy.
- Pace your activities.
- Get your family and friends to support only healthy behaviour.
- Be open and reasonable with your doctor.
- Be empathetic with others having pain problems.
- Remain hopeful.

# References

1. Frank A. Low back pain. *Br Med J* 1993; **306**: 901–9
2. Burn L. Backache in general practice. *The Practitioner* 1992; **236**: 1084–7
3. Laws D. Widening treatment dimensions for the management of low back pain. *Horizons* 1993; 362–9
4. Coste J, Delecoeuillerie G, Cohen de Lara A *et al.* (1994) Clinical course and prognostic factors in acute low back pain: an inception cohort study in primary care practice. *Br Med J* 1994; **308**: 577–80
5. Turner-Stokes L. Treatment and control of chronic arthritic and back pain. *Topical Rev Arthritis Rheumatism Council* 1993; no. 23
6. *Management of the Patient with Low Back Pain.* Physiotherapy Dept. Barnsley District General Hospital
7. Hutchinson M and Rogers R. *Moving and Lifting for Carers.* London: Woodhead Faulkner 1991
8. Halpin SFS, Yeoman L and Dundas DD. (1991) Radiographic examination of the lumbar spine in a community hospital: an audit of current practice. *Br Med J* 1991; **303**: 813–5
9. Crown S. Helping patients with persisting back pain. *Pulse* 1986; **46**: 71
10. Seers K. Chronic non malignant pain. *Br J Gen Pract* 1992; **42**: 452–3

# 6

# The management of headache in general practice

## Aims

The trainee should:

- Be able to detail an ordered and comprehensive approach to the patient who presents with a headache.
- Be able to identify those cases where there may be a serious cause for the headache.
- Be able to explain the benign nature of the non-serious causes of headache.
- Have knowledge of relieving strategies and their limitations.

## How common is headache?

Over any 2-week period, 25% of the population will have a headache severe enough to take an analgesic, and 10% will have at least one 'very severe or almost unbearable' headache each year.[1]

Some 1–2% of sufferers will present to their GP with their symptoms.[1] Of these, about 40% will have tension headache, about 30% will have migraine, and the rest will have a variety of other diagnoses.[2]

Around 20% of those presenting to the GP with headache will be referred to hospital, and headache accounts for 25% of all neurology referrals.[1] Of these, 3% will turn out to have a tumour and 5% will have specific and identifiable diseases which cause head pain, such as cranial arteritis, trigeminal neuralgia, etc. Seventy per cent will have a benign cause of their headache.[1] In around 20% a diagnosis will not be made.

The social cost of headache can be considerable. Migraine affects people of working age. It is estimated that 4 million working days are lost each year in the UK because of migraine, leading to £1200m in lost production at 1987 prices.[3]

# The causes of chronic headache

The International Headache Society classifies headache into 13 different categories. Most of these are rare and may never be encountered by a GP over a lifetime of practice. It is, however, important to be aware of their existence.

When a chronic recurring headache is presented to a GP, the most likely cause is a tension headache, closely followed by migraine. In children aged 5–15, however, migraine is commoner than tension headache.[4]

## Raised intracranial pressure

In all cases of headache it is important to exclude raised intracranial pressure and a space-occupying lesion. There is usually a progressively worsening headache. The headache typically has gradual onset and is poorly localized. Pain is worse on lying down, coughing and stooping. It often begins early in the morning and wakes the patient from sleep.

The findings of focal neurological signs or altered consciousness and papilloedema mean that you have a neurosurgical emergency on your hands, and urgent referral is needed.

Brain tumour is very rare in patients under 55 years. However, in the rare instance of a childhood tumour, headache, vomiting and ataxia or unsteadiness are particularly worrying features.

## 1. Tension headache

Tension headache is very common. The headaches may be episodic or chronic, often having been present for months or years. The typical pain is described as a 'weight on the head' or a 'tight band round the head'. There may be associated nausea, photophobia and phonophobia but actual vomiting is rare.

Exertion may relieve the symptoms. There is often no change in activity levels whatever the graphic terms in which the patient describes the severity of the symptoms.

Physical signs are usually absent. In some cases, however, the neck and shoulder muscles show increased tone, and in this group massage or other strategies to relieve the muscle tension can also relieve the headache.

Treatment response is often disappointing, one diagnostic pointer being that simple analgesia is often ineffective despite full dosage being used. A psychological approach possibly including psychotherapy, counselling and emotional support may help, but some patients will not take kindly to suggestions that their pain is psychosomatic as this will be taken as an inference that the pain is imaginary.

It is sometimes possible to detect significant psychological pathology in the course of the assessment of a tension headache, for instance a hidden depression. This will need treatment in its own right. Additionally many patients will be able through discussion to appreciate the possible role of a recent life event in the aetiology of their symptoms. Identification of such an event can make a diagnosis of tension more acceptable to the patient.

Non-steroidal anti-inflammatory drugs (NSAIDs) may help the headache more than simple analgesics. Tricyclic antidepressants in a dose of 75–150 mg/day may help, as may propranolol 30–120 mg/day, but these drugs are not licensed for this indication. Where available, biofeedback, behavioural programmes and relaxation are worth a try.[5]

Tension headache and migraine commonly coexist – a situation which used to be called combination headache. Treatment should be directed towards the most important headache for the patient, but migraine is usually easier to treat.

## 2. Migraine

Eight per cent of men and 25% of women have migraine at some stage in their lives. There is an overall community prevalence of 12%. Of these, 70% treat themselves, and of the 30% who do present their symptoms to a doctor, only a tenth are under continuing care.[6]

Typically the first attack occurs during the teens or early 20s, and it is rare for a first attack of migraine to occur over the age of 50,[5] though it is not uncommon for attacks to recur into the 40s. On average each migraine sufferer gets one attack per month.[5] The attacks often abate during middle age, but there is always a chance in the migraineur that the symptoms will restart. Peak age for attacks is 20–40.[2]

All social groups are equally affected, although there is some evidence that the higher social groups are more likely to consult with their symptoms.

*Features of migraine*
The headache of migraine may be associated with other clinical features. Not all are present in all types of migraine, but for each sufferer the pattern of symptoms will usually be the same for each

attack. Indeed, if there is a change in the pattern of the symptoms it is important to start again from basics to find out if there is another cause for the headaches.

The migraine sufferer is quite well between attacks, however severe they are. If the unwellness is persisting, this again casts doubt on the diagnosis.

*Prodrome*    This occurs for about a day before the headache, and causes subtle changes in mood or behaviour. There may be lethargy and yawning, or sometimes a feeling of extreme well-being. There may be insatiable hunger and cravings.

*Aura*    The aura consists of neurological symptoms which occur in the hour or so before the headache starts. Symptoms are typically visual (including the highly characteristic fortification spectra where objects appear to have battlement-shaped edges).

Alternatively there may be focal motor or sensory symptoms which may be very similar to those you might expect following a stroke. Such symptoms can be particularly alarming.

*Headache*    The headache of migraine is typically severe and throbbing, and lasts from 4 to 72 hours. It is accompanied by nausea or vomiting and photophobia. The pain may occur all over the head or may be localized to just one part, usually a hemisphere.

*Types of migraine*
The International Headache Society divides migraine into those with aura (about 10%, the old classical migraine), and those without aura (the old common migraine). The definitions are important as migraine treatments in general only work for true migraine. Some patients use the word migraine to describe any headache which they are finding severe.

*Migraine with aura*    The patient must have suffered at least two attacks in which a minimum of three of the following were present:[3]

- One or more fully reversible aura symptoms indicating focal cortical and/or brain dysfunction.
- At least one aura symptom developing over 4 minutes, or two or more symptoms occurring in succession.
- No aura symptoms lasting more than 60 minutes. If more than one aura symptom is present, the accepted duration is proportionately longer.
- Headache follows aura with a free interval of less than 60

minutes. It may also begin before or simultaneously with the aura.

*Migraine without aura[3]*
- A duration (untreated or unsuccessfully treated) of between 4 and 72 hours.
- At least one of the following symptoms during an attack:
  Nausea and/or vomiting.
  Photophobia and phonophobia.
- At least two of the following headache characteristics:
  Unilateral location.
  Pulsating quality.
  Moderate or severe intensity (limiting daily activities).
  Aggravated by routine physical activity.

*Treating the acute migraine attack*

*Principles of treatment[6]*
- Proprietary treatments are effective in many cases.
- If simple analgesics in preparations which also contain antiemetics are not helpful, there is little advantage in prescribing stronger ones. The patient's personal preference of analgesic is the best choice.
- Sleep can aid recovery and so it is better to avoid preparations containing caffeine, which tends to produce wakefulness.
- Oral medication should be taken as early as possible with a hot drink and a biscuit or toast, as its efficacy is impaired by gastric stasis.

*Analgesia*    Aspirin 300–900 mg (1–3 tablets) or paracetamol 500–1000 mg (1–2 tablets) every 4 hours are both effective. NSAIDs can be used, but are not licensed for this indication. The usual contraindications for aspirin and NSAIDs as far as gastric irritation is concerned should be observed.

A number of over-the-counter preparations specifically marketed to counter migraine are available. They are usually mixtures of simple analgesic plus antiemetic, and sometimes plus other things. They are generally useful, but relatively expensive when you consider what they contain.

If vomiting is a problem then indomethacin and diclofenac can be effective as suppositories.

Stronger analgesics have no advantage over simple ones in the treatment of acute migraine[16] and indeed may aggravate the overall clinical picture because they produce nausea.

*Antiemetics*    Gastric stasis is a feature of the migraine attack. Soluble medication will thus be absorbed more rapidly with increased clinical benefit.[7] For the same reason, the addition of metoclopramide or domperidone may help with the stasis, thereby curing the nausea and assisting the absorption of the analgesics. Metoclopramide is the first choice, but the chances of it causing acute extrapyramidal reactions are higher in the young and in women.

A number of migraine treatments are combinations of simple analgesia and an antiemetic. These are convenient, usually well-tolerated, and only command a single prescription charge.

*Ergot*    Ergot has been used in the treatment of migraine since 1894, and is effective in 50% of cases.[7] If used orally, bioavailability is highly variable and so the nasal, rectal or sublingual route is preferred.

Its use is dangerous in coronary heart disease, hypertension and peripheral vascular disease because of its tendency to cause arteriospasm. Similarly, concomitant use of β-blockers is contra-indicated.

A 2 mg tablet is taken as early in the attack as possible. If there is no response, another whole or half tablet is taken after 30 minutes, and this can be repeated at 30-minute intervals up to a maximum of 4 tablets.

*Ergotism* can occur at doses over 12 mg a week. A dull headache is produced which can only be abated by the next dose of ergot. The patient will need to be weaned off slowly, and this may require admission.

*Emergency treatment*    The GP is occasionally called to attend the severe migraine attack which has not responded to normal treatment. It is tempting in such circumstances to use an injection of a narcotic analgesic as the pain is so severe. Unfortunately, this will usually render the patient unfit to work for the next 24 hours, may cause habituation, and reinforces a piece of dependent health-seeking behaviour.

- Check that sufficient quantity and frequency of simple analgesia have been used.
- Troublesome vomiting can be overcome by using an antiemetic such as metoclopramide or domperidone, or conversely by using the rectal route.
- An injection of diclofenac is often useful, and will not make the patient unduly drowsy or nauseous.

- *Sumatriptan* 100 mg by injection helps over 80% of acute attacks within 15 minutes.[8] Forty per cent of responders have a recurrence within 48 hours, in which case a second injection may help. There may be a tendency for it to cause heart arrhythmias, so it should not be used in patients who might be at risk. It costs £20 per injection.

  Oral sumatriptan 300 mg is effective in 30 minutes in 65% of migraine attacks. Each tablet costs £8 and they come in packs of 6.

## The prophylaxis of migraine

Prophylactic treatment of their migraine may be preferred by patients for a number of reasons.[9] Simple analgesics take at least 2 hours to work. Ergot is toxic. Sumatriptan is too expensive for general use. No acute medication will prevent any aura, and the aura can be the most distressing aspect of an attack, especially if it involves focal neurological symptoms. Even if prophylaxis is not completely effective, it may none the less make acute treatment more likely to work.

Any prophylaxis with drugs should be tried for 3–6 months. This ensures that the treatment has had a chance to work. Also the effects of some medication, notably propranolol, often wears off after 6 months' use, but it can often be reintroduced at a later time with effect.

*Avoiding triggers*   Up to 50% of patients can help themselves by avoiding situations in which their migraine is likely to occur.[6] The link can be established by the use of a migraine diary where over a period of time the patient records any factors which might trigger an attack, and the pattern of the attacks. The migraine process starts up to 2 days before the headache emerges, so the timing of the trigger has to be right.

A number of possible triggers have been observed.[10] They are cumulative, so that one or more triggers may increase the risk of an attack to a threshold beyond which an attack results. Examples include:

- Insufficient food – missing meals, delayed meals.
- Specific foods, especially cheese, chocolate, red wine. The proportion of migraine attacks which can be attributed to specific food triggers is controversial, with some authorities claiming that most migraine is linked to food sensitivity. This view is not universally supported.
- Sleep – too little or too much.

- Environmental – bright lights, overexertion, weather.
- Hormonal – the oral contraceptive or hormone replacement therapy. If migraine with neurological symptoms occurs for the first time in somebody taking a combined oral contraceptive pill, it should be discontinued.
- Emotional stress and overwork.

*Propranolol*   Starting at a dose of 10 mg three time a day and increasing up to 120 mg a day is effective in about 60% of patients.[11] The usual contraindications should be observed, notably asthma and heart failure. Other $\beta$-blockers may also work, but they are not licensed for use in migraine.

*Pizotifen*   A nightly dose of 0.5–4.5 mg reduces attacks by 50% in 50% of migraine sufferers.[3] Drowsiness and weight gain can be problems. The chemically related methysergide is also effective, but up to 40% of recipients get retroperitoneal fibrosis, so use is restricted to hospitals.

*Clonidine*   Clonidine has a licence for use in the prophylaxis of migraine, but is no better than placebo.[3]

*Others*   Calcium channel blockers are used in many parts of the world, but are not licensed for use for migraine in the UK. They are about as effective as propranolol.

Feverfew (*Tanacetum parthenium*) is a herbal remedy which is effective, possibly because of antiprostaglandin activity. It may cause a sore tongue, dyspepsia and mouth ulcers.

Homoeopathy and acupuncture may be effective in some cases. They are probably effective but have not as yet been submitted to formal clinical evaluation.[6]

An aspirin a day may work in some patients.

Amitriptyline starting at 10 mg at night and rising to 75 mg is also effective, but migraine is not a licensed indication for its use. Depression may coexist with migraine, and this may lead to its effectiveness.

## 3.  Exotic headaches

Other non-migrainous headaches are occasionally encountered by the GP.[5] Many are quite dramatic in their presentation. If the GP has at least heard of them, the management, including reassurance, is more convincing.

## Cluster headaches

Cluster headaches are very severe unilateral head pains occurring on alternate days, up to 8 times a day, and lasting for 15 minutes to 3 hours at a time. Pains come in bouts (hence cluster) lasting several weeks with remission lasting months or years.

This is one of the few types of headache where men are affected more often than women, the ratio being 3:1.

Ipsilateral autonomic disturbance is common with facial sweating, and even Horner's syndrome (conjunctival injection, miosis and ptosis) may occur.

Treatments are not very effective. Lithium is probably the best. High-dose steroids may abort a cluster. Ergot can help. Pizotifen is not as good as methysergide. NSAIDs can help. Treatment with oxygen may help an acute attack within 10 minutes.

## Chronic paroxysmal hemicrania

Chronic paroxysmal hemicrania is different from cluster headache only in the brevity of the attacks, which last for minutes (range 3–45). They invariably resolve completely with indomethacin, which may also be used in doses of 25–100 mg a day to prevent attacks.

## Trigeminal neuralgia

Trigeminal neuralgia causes an intermittent burning pain which occurs in the distribution of the trigeminal nerve. Cold wind and eating typically aggravate the symptoms. Carbamazepine is the treatment of choice, followed by phenytoin.

## Miscellaneous headaches

This group are so obscure they don't even fit into one of the International Headache Society's 13 categories. Highlights include:

*Icepick headache or cephalalgia fugax*
These are intense head pains which last a fraction of a second only. They often occur in migraine sufferers. Indomethacin is the treatment of choice.

*External compression headache*
External compression headache results if a cutaneous cephalic nerve is compressed, for instance by swimming goggles.

*Benign exertional headache*
Benign exertional headache comes on with exercise, and is often like migraine in character. A worrying variant is associated with sexual activity. Propranolol and indomethacin often help.

*Coital cephalalgia*
Coital cephalalgia, thunderclap headache and exploding head syndrome are all of acute onset. Their first presentation will often require hospital admission.

# The causes of acute headache

The first episode of a chronic relapsing type of headache may present acutely, but patients usually wait until a few episodes have occurred before consulting.

## Infection

*Pyrexia*
Pyrexia of whatever origin can cause a headache. In particular, influenza and flu-like illness can cause headache as part of an overall body ache.

*Sinusitis*
Sinusitis is a common complication of the common cold, especially in those who have had previous episodes either because of the particular anatomy of their sinuses, or because allergic thickening of the mucosa predisposes them to the problem. The five features – a common cold, purulent rhinorrhoea, pain on bending, unilateral maxillary pain and pain in the teeth – have all been shown to correlate with ultrasonographic evidence of sinus infection.[12]

Sinusitis is uncommon in children as the maxillary sinus is only a small air cell at birth, and the frontal sinuses only start to form after the age of 6.

Treatment[13] is by broad-spectrum antibiotic such as amoxycillin or co-trimoxazole, but it may take 10 days for it to work. Steam inhalations also help the symptoms, as do decongestant nasal drops such as $\frac{1}{2}$% ephedrine.

*Bacterial meningitis*
Bacterial meningitis is characterized by a throbbing headache, but there is also systemic disturbance with fever, photophobia,

meningism and often altered conscious state. Urgent admission is needed and may be life-saving.

### Viral meningitis
Viral meningitis tends to run a milder course than its bacterial cousin.

### Encephalitis
Encephalitis may cause headache, but there is also evidence of cerebral dysfunction with confusion, clouding of consciousness and disorientation.

## Haemorrhage

### Subarachnoid haemorrhage
Subarachnoid haemorrhage usually presents very acutely and is often described by those who are able to do so as like being hit very hard on the back of the head. Sudden loss of consciousness often results and death is not infrequent. The problem is usually caused by a congenitally present aneurysm which ruptures.

Up to 60% of subarachnoid haemorrhage is preceded by one or a number of warning leaks in the month before the haemorrhage.[14] In these episodes a severe headache occurs with pain in the head or face which is often hemicranial, hemifacial or periorbital. A third-nerve palsy may occur, as may vomiting and photophobia. The presence of meningism is a particular indicator to the diagnosis.

### Posttraumatic haemorrhage
*Extradural haemorrhage*   Extradural haemorrhage is usually caused by a bleed from the middle meningeal artery. After a head injury, all is apparently well for several hours (the lucid interval) until the rapid onset of a deteriorating level of consciousness.

### Subdural haemorrhage
Subdural haemorrhage tends to occur in the elderly as brain shrinkage makes it more likely. The preceding trauma may be minor and forgotten. Several days later the bleed expresses itself as headache, fluctuating levels of consciousness and sometimes personality changes.

### Giant cell arteritis
This affects an older group of patients and is often associated with polymyalgia rheumatica. There is a temporal headache of a

persisting nature which traditionally comes to light when patients are troubled when putting on a hat or brushing their hair. Localized scalp tenderness and sometimes a cord-like and very tender cranial artery may be palpated. A raised erythrocyte sedimentation rate (ESR) is typical but not universal, and though a cranial artery biopsy may confirm the diagnosis, it is only 60–73% sensitive.[15]

The most important complication is of sudden permanent blindness if the retinal artery becomes involved.

Treatment is by oral prednisolone 20 mg a day, or 40 mg if there is ocular involvement.[15] Larger initial doses used to be used, but larger doses are associated with a greater frequency of side-effects (up to 75%) and no improvement in effectiveness. When symptomatic control is achieved (the reduction in the ESR is usually closely matched by clinical improvement), the dose can be reduced to 10 mg a day and thereafter by 1 mg a month. If the dose can be reduced to below 5 mg a day without relapse, then side-effects from the prednisolone are not troublesome.

# A consultation for headache

Consultations for headache are relatively common in general practice. Quite a lot of ground has to be covered when making an initial assessment of headache. You may as well settle in for a longish consultation.

Fears about the headache may take a little time to elicit. Many patients will be reluctant to discuss any sources of worry or stress at the outset as they do not wish their symptoms to be dismissed as being 'due to nerves' and a significant pathology thereby missed.

The assessment of headache involves physical, psychological and social dimensions. If you try and cut corners or jump to conclusions, a serious diagnosis may be missed, or patients will leave feeling dissatisfied that not only do they still have the headache, but their concerns have not been addressed either. The patient should be given sufficient time to explain the problem. It is often useful to reflect questions back, or use summaries to make sure that your understanding of the problem is consistent with the information which the patient wished to communicate.

Taking an adequate history is the mainstay of diagnosis when presented with a case of headache.

Key objectives for the GP when dealing with a patient with headache are as follows.

## Empathy

Only a minority of patients with headache will present to a doctor, so those who do present have reasons for doing so. The symptoms may be felt to be particularly severe or disruptive. There may be specific anxieties about the headache. These anxieties should be identified and dealt with.

All patients with headache should be taken seriously. It will usually be necessary at some stage in the management of the patient to offer explanations and reassurance. This will be ineffective unless patients feel that they have been listened to and a therapeutic relationship has been established.

## Exclude serious pathology

Each GP will on average encounter a new brain tumour only once every 10 years. It is important not to miss it when it does come. Other serious causes of headache are equally rare. Asking the right questions and making the right examination will ensure that nothing is missed.

Making a negative diagnosis will often not convince the patient. If a positive diagnosis can be made, this will help in the reassurance process.

## Find out why the patient has presented now

There may have been a change in or a worsening of symptoms. It is quite possible for more than one type of headache to be present. Changed symptoms may indicate a new pathological process which has to be assessed in its own right. If more than one type of headache is present, the patient will often be able to tell you the differences in symptom pattern.

## Involve the patient

The commonest type of headache, tension headache, is very resistant to treatment. You and the patient will thus be in a situation of managing chronic intractable pain. If coming to terms with such a pain is to be at all effective, the patient must retain ownership of the pain and responsibility for its effects on his or her life.

# Questions to ask[16]

1. How long has the headache been present, and have you had similar headaches in the past? A prolonged duration of

identical symptoms precludes any progressive pathological process.

2. Is the headache recurring or persistent? Migraine is episodic and there is complete relief between attacks. Tension headache is more persistent.
3. Where is the headache? Cervical spine or neck muscle problems can cause pain arising from the neck and spreading upwards. Tension headaches are usually all over the head. Migraine is frequently one-sided.
4. How long does the headache last? Migraines last a maximum of 72 hours.
5. Are there any associated symptoms? Twenty-five per cent of migraine sufferers get an aura. Neurological symptoms may be part of migraine, but the question of intracranial pathology should also be addressed.
6. Are nausea and vomiting present? Ninety-five per cent of migraine sufferers have nausea and/or vomiting (and 20% have diarrhoea). Tension headache may cause nausea but not vomiting. Effortless vomiting is associated with raised intra-cranial pressure.
7. What makes the headache better? Sleep, dark and quiet improve migraine attacks.
8. What brings the headache on?
9. What drugs are you taking? This will be an assessment of the severity of the pain, and its response to treatment. Tension headache responds poorly to analgesics. It may also point to a diagnosis of analgesic headache: if analgesics in the aspirin/paracetamol class or ergotamine are taken over the course of 3 months or more at a rate of more than three times a week[6] or more than 30 tablets a month, a headache may be caused which then only temporarily resolves with the next dose of medication.
10. Do you have any specific worries about the headache? Sometimes the headache will be disrupting work or a favoured hobby. Patients will commonly be concerned about a brain tumour, raised blood pressure or an imminent stroke. It is useful to predict some of the commoner concerns and discuss them without prompting. This has the added advantage that the patient will then believe that his or her concerns are appropriate and normal.

Concerns should be identified and discussed. Failure to do so will lead to a dissatisfied patient who is less likely to comply with any treatment, and who is likely to have symptoms aggravated by continuing worries.

## A suggested examination[3]

A clinical examination rarely reveals useful information. However, it will be expected by the patient, and contributes to the sense that the problem is being taken seriously. An examination also has medicolegal importance as a missed diagnosis can have severe repercussions.

1. Do a central nervous system examination including cranial nerves and fundi, but remember that papilloedema is only found in around 50% of cases of brain tumour.[7]
2. Check movements of the cervical spine and temporomandibular joints.
3. Apply gentle pressure to the sinuses, and also the temporal arteries in the over-50s.
4. Auscultate the carotid arteries.
5. Measure the blood pressure. Except with very high levels, raised blood pressure does not cause headache. However, this is not commonly appreciated. Checking the blood pressure ensures that a thorough assessment job has been done, and is also a good way of opportunistic screening.

## Which cases of headache need referral?

In a number of instances, a case will be referred for a specialist opinion. The symptom of headache can generate much anxiety in patient and GP. Most of those referred will turn out to have benign problems only.

### Patient-initiated

1. Symptoms not controlled.
2. Diagnosis in doubt or in dispute.

### GP-initiated

1. Symptoms refractory to treatment.
2. Possible analgesic abuse.
3. Diagnosis in doubt.

## Sinister symptoms

1. Recent onset of severe headache, especially in the over-50s.
2. Morning headache on waking, plus vomiting.
3. Progressively more severe headaches.
4. Neurological deficit or seizure.
5. Complicated migraine, for instance hemiplegic migraine.
6. Papilloedema suspected.
7. Possible subarachnoid haemorrhage.
8. Known malignancy or endocrine dysfunction.

# References

1. Lane RJM. Is it migraine? The differential diagnosis. *Update* 1991; **43**: 760–74
2. Fowler TJ. Management of headache. *Update* 1991; **43**: 635–53
3. Hackett G. Management of migraine. *The Practitioner* 1994; **238**: 130–6
4. Abu-Arefeh I & Russell G. Prevalence of headache and migraine in schoolchildren. *Br Med J* 1994; **309**: 765–9
5. Clough C. Non-migrainous headaches. *Br Med J* 1989; **299**: 70–2
6. MacGregor EA. Prescribing for migraine. *Prescribers' J* 1993; **33**: 50–8
7. Kenny C. Headaches and migraines. *Horizons* 1992; **6**: 430–33
8. Sumatriptan: a new approach to migraine. *Drug Ther Bull* 1992; **30**: 85–87
9. Peatfield R & Beaumont G. Migraine prophylaxis. *Med Dialogue* No 370. 1992; pp 1–4
10. MacGregor A. Make sure the symptoms point clearly to migraine. *Horizons* 1993; **7**: 390–4
11. Gambrill E. Symptomatic treatment of headache. *Update* 1993; **47**: 239–44
12. van Duijn NP, Brouwer HJ & Lamberts H. Use of symptoms and signs to diagnose maxillary sinusitis in general practice: comparison with ultrasonography. *Br Med J* 1992; **305**: 684–7
13. Johnston D & Gleeson M. Maxillary sinusitis. *The Practitioner* 1993; **237**: 297–302
14. Ostergaard JR. Warning leak in subarachnoid haemorrhage. *Br Med J* 1990; **301**: 190–1
15. Mason JC & Walport MJ. Giant cell arteritis. *Br Med J* 1992; **305**: 68–9
16. Wilkinson M. Management of headache. *The Practitioner* 1992; **236**: 449–51

# 7

# Premenstrual syndrome (PMS)

## Aims

The trainee should:

- Know the symptomatic manifestations of PMS.
- Be able to empathize with the patient presenting with PMS.
- Be aware of the therapeutic options available and their limitations.

## What is PMS?

Premenstrual tension was first described in 1931, and later the definition was widened to PMS to include the non-psychological features of the disorder.

PMS has been defined as 'distressing physical and psychological symptoms, not caused by organic disease, which regularly recur during the same phase of each menstrual (or ovarian) cycle, and which significantly regress or disappear during the remainder of the cycle'.[1]

This definition emphasizes the two cardinal features of PMS:

- Symptoms occur during the luteal phase of the menstrual cycle and resolve completely by the end of menstruation.[2] There must be at least 7 days of the menstrual cycle free of symptoms.[3] The typical pattern is for symptoms to build up during the 7–10 days before the menses begin, to be at a maximum the day before menstruation, and then resolve within a few days thereafter. Some women also experience symptoms at midcycle just before ovulation.[4]
- The symptoms are sufficiently severe to interfere appreciably with normal functioning or interpersonal relationships.

Around 150 different symptoms have been ascribed to PMS,[3] so the type of symptom is not specific. It is the timing of the symptoms which distinguishes PMS. Some commoner symptoms are:

**Emotional and behavioural**

- Depression.
- Irritability.
- Lability.
- Anxiety
- Loss of self-control.
- Poor concentration.
- Change in libido.
- Aggression or violence.
- Food cravings.
- Fatigue.

**Physical**

- Headache.
- Breast swelling.
- Breast tenderness.
- Backache.
- Weight gain.
- Abdominal bloating.
- Acne.
- Swollen fingers and ankles.
- Gastrointestinal disturbances.

# What is not PMS?

The symptoms of PMS are not specific, and are found widely in the male as well as the female population. Indeed, the vast majority of the general population will have some of the symptoms some of the time. A common reason for such symptoms is a depressive disorder, or a reaction to adverse social circumstances or life events. Depression is often accompanied by guilt and stigma so that patients may be hoping to pin an 'acceptable' diagnosis of PMS on their symptoms rather than contemplate the possibility of a depressive illness.

It is not uncommon for women to present at the surgery saying at the outset that they think they have PMS, and asking what can be done about it. At this stage it is necessary to establish the correct diagnosis firmly before rational management can proceed. As will be seen, the treatments available for PMS do not always work, and they certainly will not work if the patient is not suffering from PMS in the first place.

Three other categories of symptoms should be distinguished from PMS:[2]

1. Physiological premenstrual symptoms occur at the right time but are not severe enough to constitute PMS.
2. Psychiatric disorders wrongly attributed to PMS. Many symptoms of depression are the same as those of PMS, and are often confused.
3. Secondary PMS occurs when an underlying physical or psychological disturbance is responsible for the symptoms. Symptoms improve but do not completely resolve after menses. This is also sometimes called menstrual distress. However, PMS may be superimposed on to other problems, in which case treating the PMS may partially help.

## How common is PMS?

Premenstrual symptoms occur in 95% of women of reproductive age.[21] Around 30% have symptoms sufficiently severe to consult their doctor.[3] Five per cent of women are severely incapacitated,[2, 3] and some are so badly affected that there are suicides, parasuicides and attempted acts of violence against others.

## Who gets PMS?

Women of any age from the menarche to the menopause may be affected, but the commonest age is the third and fourth decades.[5] Sufferers are often affected for the whole of their reproductive lives, though symptoms may fluctuate in severity. Parity does not affect symptoms.[3] The only reliable end to symptoms is the cessation of ovulation by biological, chemical or surgical means.[2]

## What causes PMS?

The cause of PMS is unknown.

There may be a genetic component, as concordance for PMS between monozygotic twins is more than for dizygotic twins.

It is suggested that neuroticism and poor self-image are associated with PMS,[5] but this remains unproven.[3]

Salt and water retention as a cause has also recently been discounted.[2]

PMS does not occur when the normal cycle of sex hormone changes is abolished, so there must be a hormonal factor involved. However, sufferers from PMS do not differ from others with respect to hormone levels, so it is the fluctuations in levels rather than the hormones themselves which are implicated.

A number of substances mediate sex hormone effects on neurotransmitter functions in the brain. Included in these are β-endorphin and serotonin; PMS sufferers have lower levels of both of these during the luteal phase.[2]

Women need more sleep in the premenstrual days,[6] and so it is suggested that lack of sleep may contribute to the symptoms of PMS.

Some symptoms of PMS are similar to those of hypoglycaemia. Though it has not been confirmed that PMS sufferers do have chronic or recurrent low blood sugar, this theory has suggested another treatment approach.

Many other factors have a role in the development of PMS symptoms.[2] They include environmental, psychosocial and personal factors such as stress, interpersonal relationship problems, underlying psychopathology and problems with personality, self-esteem and general health and well-being.

## How to make the diagnosis

Premenstrual symptoms are very common among women of ovulating age. Retrospective assessment of symptoms has been shown in a number of studies to overestimate incidence and severity. A more accurate assessment of the problem can be achieved prospectively by the use of a symptom diary for a minimum of 2 months.[7]

There are no reliable investigations for PMS. It has been suggested that erythrocyte magnesium levels are consistently lower in PMS sufferers,[2] and these levels can be measured.

Goserelin is a gonadotrophin-releasing hormone analogue. Two months' treatment will suppress genuine PMS symptoms completely. A 3-month trial is given, and if there has not been a resolution or improvement of symptoms by the third month, then the symptoms are not due to PMS. This can be used as a diagnostic test, but its use should be confined to hospital practice.

## What can the GP do? Management plan

### Empathy

In many cases the symptoms of PMS are very disruptive and

troublesome, and the GP should take them seriously. Talking through what is happening and a discussion of the possible reasons for the symptoms may be all that the woman wants.

A placebo rate of at least 50% and up to 94% is reported in studies on the treatment of PMS.[3] This may reflect the important benefits to be gained from a sympathetic approach, and the fact that attention is being paid to the problem. For milder physiological symptoms, drug treatment is rarely successful.

When considering treatment options it is important to establish the patient's agenda. What are the priorities for treatment? What are the main symptoms from which relief is sought? What sorts of treatment would be acceptable? What treatments have already been tried?

The only treatments which can be relied upon to abolish PMS symptoms completely are those which suppress ovulation, which is clearly no good for someone who wishes a pregnancy.

## Make sure it's PMS

Physical causes of similar symptoms should be excluded. Myxoedema, ovarian cyst and endometriosis are worth particular consideration and will need managing appropriately. Dysmenorrhoea and climacteric symptoms may present as PMS.

Psychological pathology such as depression and panic disorder may be suspected. Suitable open-ended questions and a receptive attitude may help. Up to 25% of depressed patients present with physical symptoms, but in only 9% are there no psychological symptoms at all,[8] so in a majority of cases, even if a physical problem is the primary presentation, some psychological symptoms are also identifiable.

Social factors such as relationship problems, debt and deprivation may be associated with PMS-type symptoms. On the other hand, PMS may cause these problems. At least one charge of murder in the UK has been successfully defended on the grounds that the killer was suffering from PMS at the time.

A diary of symptoms will confirm the cyclical nature of the symptoms. Suitable diary sheets are obtainable from the Women's Nutritional Advisory Service and the Consumers' Association. These have space for the symptoms which that individual has, and a three-point scale of the severity of them day by day. This is matched with another column in which the days of menses are noted. After 2 months' use it should be possible to confirm or refute the relationship of symptoms to the menstrual cycle.

## Non-drug treatments

### Psychological approaches

Psychological approaches include counselling, stress management and cognitive therapy. They are all time-consuming and/or costly in terms of qualified professional input. Some women will be unwilling or unable to participate in such treatments. Effects are difficult to quantify.

### Complementary advice

Complementary medical advice may be sought in the form of yoga, acupuncture or hypnosis.

### Diet[9]

Some of the various theories on the cause of PMS have suggested a dietary approach to treatment. Luckily the recommendations are in most important respects identical to general advice for a healthy diet.

- Reduce the intake of sugar and 'junk' foods. Sugars cause a rebound hypoglycaemia.
- Reduce the amount of salt. This includes added salt and salt in cooking or processing. Palatability may become a problem.
- Reduce tea and coffee intake. Too much caffeine causes irritability.
- Limit the intake of animal fats.
- Use good-quality vegetable oils and margarines. This increases polyunsaturated fat intake.
- Limit the use of alcohol and tobacco – cigarettes to 5 a day, alcohol to 7 units a week.
- Eat plenty of nutritious wholesome foods. Vegetables are better than fruits, and bran may block the absorption of other nutrients.
- Eat regularly. A meal or snack every 3 hours avoids hypoglycaemia.
- Lose weight if you are obese.
- Be patient. Treatment may take up to 3 months to work.

### Dietary supplements[2]

- Pyridoxine (vitamin $B_6$) is probably worth a try. The dose is 100–200 mg/day throughout the cycle. Smaller doses have no proven effect,[5] and doses over 500 mg a day may cause peripheral neuropathy.
- Magnesium and Calcium supplements may help. These are both

involved in neurotransmitter synthesis, so their use is at least logical.
- Evening primrose oil has fervent advocates, and may be worth trying. Its only licensed indication for PMS symptoms is, however, for cyclical mastalgia, so it cannot be prescribed when cyclical mastalgia is absent from the symptom pattern. It can be bought but in its recommended dose of 3–4 capsules twice a day for the full cycle it is rather expensive.

## Lifestyle[9]

- When under stress, take time to relax each day.
- Communicate with your partner and family. If you have symptoms they should be warned. They may even want to help.
- Get a good night's sleep. Patients with PMS need more sleep.[6]
- Take care when making difficult decisions premenstrually. Women who have undertaken criminal acts are more likely to get caught by the police in the 2 premenstrual weeks.
- Keep up to date with jobs at home and at work.
- Take regular physical exercise. Improving general fitness may make PMS symptoms more bearable. The resulting increase in endorphins may help psychological symptoms.

## Medication

The wide range of tablet treatments suggested reflects the various theories on the aetiology of PMS. This indicates that none of them are particularly good, and this is confirmed by research data. Most studies have in any case been performed by pharmaceutical manufacturers in pursuit of their own particular ends, and have often involved small numbers of patients.[2]

### Non-hormone medication

- Clomipramine and fluoxetine have both been shown in trials to be effective for the psychological symptoms of primary and secondary PMS.
- Bromocriptine 2.5 mg at night will help in mastalgia.
- Spironolactone 100 mg/day for the second half of the cycle will help in fluid retention, but only when this has been confirmed by weight gain. It is no good for abdominal bloating without weight gain.
- Mefenamic acid 250–500 mg three times daily from day 16 to day 3 can be helpful for fatigue, irritability, aches and pains and mood symptoms. Other non-steroidal anti-inflammatory drugs probably work as well.

*Hormones*

Only progesterone, progestagens and bromocriptine have a specific licence for use in PMS.

- Dydrogesterone 10 mg twice a day from days 12 to 26 has limited evidence for its usefulness generally in PMS.
- Progesterone in the form of pessaries and suppositories is widely used, but there is no evidence from controlled trials that it is effective.[2]
- Oestrogens have a proven effect when given by patches and implants.[3] Since they suppress ovulation, their efficacy is logical. The additional progestagens which have to be given cyclically to avoid endometrial hyperplasia will in 50% of cases cause symptoms to restart,[2] but they are often different from the original crop of symptoms. The benefits of treatment may decay with time.

The oral contraceptive pill may also be effective, but in some patients it will actually increase symptoms. It may be given continuously if the usual cyclical regime is ineffective.

*Other treatments*

The above will normally be the extent that the average GP will wish to become involved with PMS treatment. Specialized clinics may wish to pursue further treatment options.

- *Danazol*

Danazol suppresses ovulation very effectively and thus relieves PMS. Side-effects are common at the higher doses of 400 mg/day and include weight gain, acne and hirsutism. Doses of 200 mg/day or below give fewer side-effects.

- *Goserelin*

Goserelin and other gonadotrophin-releasing hormone analogues work in severe PMS, but cause hot flushes, atrophic vaginitis and osteoporosis with long-term use. They are very expensive.

- *Surgery*

Surgery may be needed in severe cases. Oophorectomy will abolish symptoms, and hysterectomy alone may help as it modifies ovarian activity. Very occasionally, hysterectomy is needed to obviate the need for progestagens in oestrogen therapy.

## Choosing the right treatment

The aim of treatment should be to remove or render tolerable the symptoms by the simplest means. Patient characteristics will determine the treatment recommended. Lifestyle and dietary advice have the fewest side-effects, even though they may be the hardest type of treatment to keep to as far as the patient is concerned. All patients with PMS should be offered lifestyle and dietary advice, especially as the advice is also suitable for the general promotion of health.

The older woman approaching the menopause is a candidate for oestrogen therapy.

For women who wish a pregnancy, treatment with oestrogen, the combined oral contraceptive and anything else which suppresses ovulation is clearly inappropriate. Some treatments are also potentially teratogenic, for instance the possible masculinization of the female fetus caused by danazol.

Women with primarily psychological symptoms will benefit most from a sympathetic approach and the use of non-invasive treatments. The use of clomipramine and fluoxetine can be considered.

Women with severe symptoms which do not respond to treatment will need to be referred. The local gynaecology department can give advice, and also provide access to surgical or other interventions not available in primary care. It may be appropriate to refer women with overtly psychological symptoms to the psychiatry services. In such cases the community psychiatric nurses or counsellors (if available) can provide important support for the patient.

## What do GPs actually do?

A survey undertaken by the Women's Nutritional Advisory Service[9] showed that only pyridoxine and synthetic and natural progestagens were used by more than 50% of GPs in the treatment of PMS. A total of 27.5% gave lifestyle counselling, and 15.8% made dietary recommendations, though 92% of the group admitted no formal nutritional training.

## References

1. Magos A & Studd JWW. The premenstrual syndrome. In: Studd J (ed) *Progress in Obstetrics and Gynaecology*, vol. 4. London: Churchill Livingstone. 1984; pp. 334–50

2. O'Brien PMS. Helping women with premenstrual syndrome. *Br Med J* 1993; **307**: 1471–5
3. Managing the premenstrual syndrome. *Drug Ther Bull* 1992; **30**: 334–50
4. Smith R & Studd J. Premenstrual syndrome. *Update* 1994; **48**: 939–47
5. Scott A & Crowder AM. Premenstrual syndrome. *Update* 1993; **47**: 459–63
6. Lee S. *Learning to Cope with PMT – An Information Leaflet for Women with Premenstrual Symptoms.* Sheffield: Northern Hormone Service. 1992
7. Gath D & Iles S. Treating the premenstrual syndrome. *Br Med J* 1988; **297**: 237–8
8. Wright AF. *Depression: Recognition and Management in General Practice* London: Royal College of General Practitioners. 1993
9. Stewart A. *A Rational Approach to Treating Premenstrual Syndrome.* Hove: Women's Nutritional Advisory Service. 1989

# 8

# Painful knees

## Aims

The trainee should:

- Be able to conduct an examination of the knee.
- Know of the common causes of knee pain.
- Be able to advise appropriately on simple therapeutic regimes for knee pain.

## How common is knee trouble?

The average GP with 2000 patients should expect to see 30–40 patients with knee conditions each year. Most patients will present because of pain.[1]

Ligament and meniscal tears are common in players of contact sports such as rugby and soccer. Jumpers, such as basketball and badminton players, are prone to problems with the patellar tendon – the so-called jumper's knee. Keen athletes are particularly reluctant to undergo treatments which involve prolonged rest or a change of activity.

One in 6 girls and 1 in 14 boys suffer from anterior knee pain at some time in their lives.[1]

## Which knee structures can cause pain?

Almost any part of the knee joint can cause symptoms. Each individual structure can give rise to pain. In addition, problems may be caused by difficulty with the movements of the joint. The knee is basically a hinge joint, but in the last 10–15° of extension the lateral side of the tibia subluxes forward, which locks the knee by tightening the cruciate ligaments. The inability of a knee to hinge or lock straight can also cause symptoms.

The knee is a synovial joint involving the femur, tibia and the patella, which is a sesamoid bone of the quadriceps tendon. There are four ligaments: medial collateral from femur to tibia, lateral collateral from femur to fibular head, and anterior and posterior cruciates connecting the gaps between the two articular surfaces on each of the femur and tibia.

There are medial and lateral menisci between the femur and tibia. Each sits on its own articular surface, and is shaped like a crescent. The most important muscle is the quadriceps femoris which, as the name indicates, has four parts: the vastus medialis and lateralis, and the rectus femoris which all connect to the patella, and the iliotibial tract which runs laterally to the tibial head.

## What do you need to know?

Taking a good history can get you a long way towards establishing a diagnosis. The two most important pieces of information are:

• Has there been an injury? If so, what exactly happened?
• How old is the patient?

### If there has been an injury

Twisting of the flexed knee suggests meniscal tear. Other sports injuries suggest ligament problems, as does a feeling of the knee coming out of joint.

• Could the patient walk after the injury? Inability suggests complete ligament rupture.
• How bad is the pain? Complete ligament tears cause very little pain. After a meniscal tear it is often possible to carry on with the game as symptoms only worsen when the swelling has come up.
• Is there swelling? Swelling coming up in the 2 hours after the injury is usually due to bleeding into the joint – a haemarthrosis. Such an injury indicates severe intra-articular damage and needs referring to the local casualty department. Swelling coming up over a couple of days is usually an effusion due to more minor damage, and so there is more scope for conservative treatment.
• Has the knee given way? This may indicate an anterior cruciate rupture, a meniscal tear or a loose body in the joint.

### If there has not been an injury

• Pain on walking up or down stairs or hills, or on prolonged sitting suggests patellofemoral pathology.

- Vague diffuse pain may indicate referred pain from the hip.
- A history of injury in the past will suggest the possibility of a degenerative disorder.
- Pain and stiffness in other joints may point to generalized osteoarthritis or one of the other polyarthropathies, such as rheumatoid arthritis.

## How should you examine the knee?

In the acutely painful posttraumatic knee it may be impossible, because of pain, swelling or distortion of the knee anatomy, to make a proper examination.

### Look

- Swelling may be generalized as a result of effusion or haemarthrosis, or localized, suggesting a bursitis. Mild effusions are detected by the patellar tap or by demonstrating movement of fluid from one side of the patella to the other.
- Quadriceps wasting may be visible in any chronic knee problem.

### Feel

- Tenderness may be localized to a small area, which will help identify which structure is causing the pain.
- Tenderness on the underside of the patella when pushed sideways with the knee relaxed suggests a patellofemoral problem.

### Move

There should be a full range of movement from 0 to about 145° of flexion.

- The usual reason for reduced flexion is fluid in the joint.
- A block to extension is a locked knee and urgent referral for arthroscopy is indicated.

### Special tests

- Collateral ligaments can only be tested in 15° or more of flexion, otherwise the cruciate ligaments lock the joint. Varus and valgus strain tests the lateral and medial ligaments respectively.
- Cruciates can be checked with the draw test. With the knee at 90°

and the foot held, forward and backward force on the upper tibia tests the anterior and posterior cruciate ligaments respectively.

- Various tests for meniscal tears have been devised. They are universally sadistic in execution. Apley, the inventor of one of the tests, no longer uses it because of the pain caused.[2] The best guide to meniscal tear is:

> The nature of injury.
> The presence of an effusion.
> The presence of quadriceps wasting.
> Joint line tenderness.

## Which cases need referral?

Many cases of knee pain can be managed in general practice. Even if a definitive diagnosis is not made, it is often possible to suggest general measures to improve symptoms. In some circumstances, however, it is inappropriate for the GP to try and manage the situation:

- Possible septic arthritis. There will be an inflamed and painful joint, systemic disturbance and pyrexia. Urgent hospital treatment is required. In medicolegal terms, taking the temperature is of importance.
- Possible neoplasm. Tumours of the knee structures are very rare, but just occasionally a tumour in the femur or upper tibia will present as knee pain.
- Severe disorder. If a haemarthrosis is suspected, or there is evidence of a complete ligament tear, or if the knee is locked, then prompt referral through the local accident department is appropriate.

## Anterior knee pain

The patient is usually an active sporting adolescent who complains of knee pain, particularly at the start of exercise, and on walking up or down stairs.

### Chondromalacia patellae

This is the commonest cause of anterior knee pain. The articular cartilage on the patella becomes soft. This releases enzymes, causing pain and venous engorgement. Sometimes it is associated with maltracking of the patella so that the patella moves laterally when the knee is flexed.

The diagnosis can be made by examining the extended and supported knee. The patella can be moved sideways and the underneath palpated. Tenderness to palpation is consistent with the diagnosis.

Chondromalacia patellae is usually a self-limiting condition, but it may last up to 8 years. In 87% of cases the pain is not severe enough to have to use analgesia, but 17% have to restrict their sporting activities because of it.[1]

Analgesics, non-steroidal anti-inflammatory drugs (NSAIDs) and rest from aggravating activities are needed. If there is evidence of maltracking, quadriceps exercises can be beneficial, as can specialized strapping techniques which pull the patella medially. Physiotherapists are very good at this.

Opinion is divided, but some orthopaedic surgeons advocate a more proactive approach with arthroscopy and surgical removal of the entire cartilage. Evidence of benefit over less invasive techniques is limited.

### Osgood–Schlatter's disease

A tender swelling is found over the tibial tuberosity. The patient is usually an adolescent male who is very active and sporting. There is a typical appearance on X-ray. The condition is usually self-limiting, and the only restriction need be to avoid aggravating activities.

### Bursitis

Bursitis can affect the prepatellar bursa (housemaid's knee), or the infrapatellar bursa (clergyman's knee). There is often a history of trauma or repeated kneeling. The swelling is very localized, and may be tender but is often merely uncomfortable.

Treatment is by compressing the area with strapping and the use of an NSAID. A large bursa can be aspirated through a wide-bore needle, which also has the advantage of confirming the diagnosis and creating the satisfying impression that you have done something useful. A small amount of steroid injected into the bursa can aid resolution.

### Referred pain from the hip

A vague pain in the knee which is hard for the patient to pinpoint may indicate that the pain is arising from the hip joint. There are no signs to be found in the knee joint itself. The possibility of hip pathology should be remembered in any patient who presents with knee pain. The old axiom applies whereby the joints above and below the site of symptoms should be examined.

### Meniscal tears

A torn cartilage is an occasional surprise finding at arthroscopy for anterior knee pain. The tear should be dealt with on its merits.

### Synovial plicae

These are folds of synovial membrane that become trapped between femur and tibia on flexion. Their existence was only established when arthroscopy became widely available, but their removal sometimes secures clinical improvement.

## Acute knee injury

An acute knee injury will follow either a fall or a sporting mishap, particularly with contact sports. Keen athletes are often independent, introverted, self-reliant and self-confident.[3] These attributes will make them mistrust doctors, and they will often have taken advice from a number of other sources before they are seen by the medical services.

The injury will mean that the patient is unable to pursue his or her chosen sport, which may mean letting down other members of the team or being criticized by an overzealous coach or parent. Rehabilitation is interfered with by the desire to make up lost training time, and there may be unrealistic expectations of a solution to the injury and a quick return to the sport.

Some athletes will be injury-prone despite good technique and proper equipment. Most bodies are simply not physiologically capable of the effort and training required to be a top-class athlete.

### Acute management

The acute management of the injured knee does not require a definitive diagnosis. A large portion of these cases will self-refer to the casualty department where they will often get little sympathy for their self-inflicted injury. Often the swelling and stiffness develop gradually so that it is a day or two after the injury before the extent of the problem is appreciated.

In the acute phase proper assessment is impossible and cruel. A sudden onset of swelling suggests haemarthrosis so that major knee damage is probable: such cases need urgent referral.

The less severe case can be helped by RICE:

- R is for *rest*. This will not be a problem if the patient is having trouble walking.
- I is for *ice*. Ice packs should be applied to the joint for 10–15 minutes as often as tolerated. Bags of frozen peas or marbles are good substitutes and can be reused.
- C is for *compression*. Crepe bandage, tubular bandage or even a Robert Jones bandage will squeeze out any effusion and limit movement.
- E is for *elevation*. This also helps reduce the effusion.

### Rehabilitation

After this initial treatment, when the knee becomes more comfortable, the emphasis changes to retrieving function. After as little as 48 hours (but usually a week in patients who are not too concerned to return to their sport with the minimum delay), it will be possible to encourage movement. The physiotherapist can help with this, but where not available, passive exercises should be started. Swimming is an excellent means of doing this as the limb is supported by the water while the knee is exercised.

The use of specific exercises to retain the strength of the quadriceps muscle is an important part of rehabilitation.

### Quadriceps wasting

Quadriceps power is essential for the stability of the knee joint and the proper tracking of the patella. Unfortunately, within a few days of a knee injury which reduces function, wasting can be detected. Vastus medialis is particularly vulnerable, and weakness here can lead to lateral tracking of the patella and even dislocation.

Quadriceps bulk can often be assessed visually. However, the standard way is to measure the girth of the thigh at a point 6 cm above the top of the patella. A difference of more than 1 cm is significant.[1] Remember that muscle bulk is usually slightly greater on the dominant side.

Exercises to increase quadriceps power can be suggested for:

- Pre-sport training to avoid injury.
- Knee injuries after the acute phase is passed.

- Almost any chronic knee problem. There are a number of Premier Division professional soccer players who play with no effective cruciates, with stability being maintained just by muscle power.[2]

The basic *exercise* is straight leg raising with the foot dorsiflexed.

1. Lying down, the leg is slowly lifted to a slow count of 5.
2. The leg is held up for a count of 10.
3. The leg is slowly lowered again for a count of 5.
4. After a brief rest, the process is repeated 10 times.

This exercise can be done every hour if possible, or less frequently (or with fewer repetitions) in the less fit.

A further refinement is to put a weight on the foot, but this may lead to incomplete extension and it is the last few degrees of extension which exercise the vastus medialis.

## Meniscal tear

The typical injury which tears the meniscus is the twist to the partially flexed knee. It is thus a characteristic injury of footballers and rugby players. After the injury the player may well be able to continue the game, and it is only as the effusion builds up that it becomes apparent that something is seriously amiss. Meniscal tears may therefore not present acutely.

Having obtained the typical history, there will be the clinical findings of swelling and joint line tenderness. It is usually the medial meniscus which is torn, and so tenderness is on the medial joint line. At late presentation quadriceps wasting may also be seen.

There may be additional history that the knee has locked or given way. When a knee gives way it is most alarming as it can happen without warning and feels as though the leg has suddenly disappeared (personal observation).

X-rays are often not helpful, but magnetic resonance imaging can give useful evidence and may avoid arthroscopy. If a tear is suspected and is continuing to cause problems, then an orthopaedic opinion is required. This is not needed in all cases, as the symptoms may be so mild or infrequent that they do not cause much trouble. In the days when the full meniscectomy was the only treatment option, it was tempting to leave well alone.

Referred cases will usually proceed to arthroscopy. Under a general anaesthetic, an incision is made at either side of the patella, and fluid introduced into the joint. Afterwards the knee is heavily bandaged for a few days to disperse the fluid. Time off work depends on the job, but sedentary workers need a couple of days only while manual workers may need 2–4 weeks.

Small meniscal tears can usually be managed by arthroscopic meniscectomy where the damaged bit of cartilage is trimmed off. This is an improvement over the old open meniscectomy where the whole meniscus was removed. Removal of the entire meniscus causes disruption to joint loading, and subsequent osteoarthritis is unavoidable. Recovery from arthroscopic surgery is also quicker, though it may take 2 or 3 months until a manual worker is able to return to work.

## Osteoarthritis

About half the adult population have X-ray evidence of osteo-arthritis (OA),[4] and this rises to be an almost universal finding in the elderly.[5] There is, however, little correlation between X-ray findings and symptoms and only 1 in 8 patients aged over 65 has symptomatic OA.[5]

OA is not simply a matter of 'wear and tear' of the joint, as the process of OA is a dynamic one. There is destruction of the cartilage with chondrocyte death. In the bone, there is proliferation with subchondral sclerosis and osteophyte formation. There is hypertrophy of the ligaments and capsule, and the synovium often shows mild inflammatory changes. Varying degrees of muscle wasting also occur.

Factors predisposing to OA are:[5]

- The ageing of connective tissue.
- An inherited predisposition – a very important factor in some patients.
- Abnormal joint loading. This may be through abnormal use, or normal use in a distorted joint (such as following meniscectomy).
- Obesity.
- Female gender.

### Symptoms

Pain is the prime symptom. Cartilage has no nerve fibres, so the pain arises from other structures. It is worse on loading the joint, and worse as the day goes on. Rest relieves the pain. Stiffness is common, lasting around 30 minutes after getting up in the morning, or longer if it follows a rest in the day. The joint may 'crack', and crepitus may be found.

Pain and loss of movement both contribute to the consequent disability. The formation of osteophytes may restrict movement in the joint.

Symptoms may be persistent or intermittent. It is not unusual for an arthritic knee to start giving symptoms for no very obvious reason. This may lead the GP to think that an inflammatory arthritis is present.

## Non-drug treatment

This should always be considered first, and as an addition to other treatments.

1. Weight loss in the obese.
2. Mobility exercises. Swimming is very helpful.
3. Strength exercises will improve muscle tone, improve function and help reduce pain. The physiotherapist will advise. Exercising an arthritic knee will accelerate the radiological deterioration, but improve the symptoms.[6]
4. Aids such as splints, walking sticks. For patellofemoral OA, relief can be obtained by taping the patella medially.[7]

## Medication

The choice is between analgesics and NSAIDs. Paracetamol in a dose of 1 g four times a day is more effective than an NSAID.[5] Inflammation is not a significant component of OA, so the effectiveness of treatment depends only on analgesic power. When it is considered that NSAIDs can increase the incidence of a gastrointestinal bleed up to five-fold,[5] and that the elderly are more at risk, then this demotes the NSAIDs to definite second-line status.

In addition, there remain some concerns that NSAIDs may actually accelerate cartilage loss. This is probably true of indomethacin, but the evidence for other NSAIDs is lacking.[4]

Intra-articular steroid injections can bring fast – if short-lasting – relief. There is still controversy as to whether injecting steroid into weight-bearing joints accelerates the loss of cartilage.[4,5]

## Surgery

A knee replacement should be considered when there is pain and/or loss of function unresponsive to conservative measures including analgesia, NSAIDs, rest, physiotherapy, weight loss, a light knee splint and quadriceps-building exercises.[8] The patellofemoral joint endures five times the weight of the body when the patient is walking upstairs.[8] Because of the strength of the materials used in the prosthesis, knee replacement should be restricted to patients weighing under 80 kg.

The aim of knee replacement is to reduce pain, correct any valgus or varus deformity and to ensure proper tracking of the patella. The patient should be able to flex the knee to 110° after surgery, which is sufficient to climb stairs, drive a car, kneel down, and get on and off a bus or train.

Infection occurs in 0.5–2% of cases, and needs vigorous treatment. Some surgeons suggest the early use of antibiotics in all types of infection following prosthesis to ensure there is no spread to the knee.

Well over 90% of knee replacements last over 10 years,[8] though this is reduced in the younger patients who presumably use them more. They are thus as successful as hip replacement. Knee prostheses are also easier to revise than hips.

A knee prosthesis costs £500–£1500 (1992 figures), with some of the cheaper types giving the best long-term results.[8]

With the increased popularity of knee prostheses, other types of surgical intervention are less common. However, some patients will derive benefit from surgery to alter the loading on the joint to relieve badly affected parts.

# References

1. Jessop J. Management of anterior knee pain. *Med Monitor* 1992; **5**: 76–80
2. Hackney R & Wilson N. Knee problems. *GP Newspaper* May 1 1992; 41–4
3. Jaques RD. Management of sports injuries. *Update* 1994; **48**: 459–67
4. Jones A & Doherty M. Osteoarthritis, cartilage and NSAIDs. *Care Elderly* 1992; **4**: 97–8
5. Osteoarthritis and its treatment. *MeReC Bull* 1994; **5**:
6. Massardo L, Wall I, Cushnaghan J *et al.* Osteoarthritis of the knee joint; an 8-year prospective study. *Ann Rheum Dis* 1989; **48**(11): 893–97
7. Cushnaghan J, McCarthy C & Dieppe P. Taping the patella medially: a new treatment for osteoarthritis of the knee joint? *Br Med J* 1994: **308**: 753–5
8. Hip and knee joint replacements. *Drug Thera Bull* 1992; **30**: 57–60

# 9

# Alcohol abuse

## Aims

The trainee should:

- Be aware of the signs and symptoms of alcohol abuse.
- With the family and other health professionals, be able to construct a care programme for the alcohol-damaged patient.
- Have knowledge of the interventions available, and be able to implement them.
- Be able to advise a patient on how to reduce consumption of alcohol.

## A bit of history

The consumption of alcohol has been an important part of social life for thousands of years. The first recorded brewing was in 5000 BC when beer was part of the daily wages of the temple workers in Mesopotamia. William Pitt the Younger is alleged to have drunk 574 bottles of claret, 854 of madeira and 2410 of port in one year.

Average alcohol consumption in the UK has been rising since the 1940s following a previous decline. Consumption was about the same in terms of quantity of pure alcohol per head of population in 1980 as it was in 1900.[1]

In general, the consumption of spirits has fallen and the consumption of wine has markedly increased. In 1700 beer consumption per head was about 10 times what it was in 1980.[1]

The increase in all alcohol consumption over the last 25 years has been most marked in women and in the 18–25-year age group.[2] The cost of alcohol is coming down. For a man on an average wage, in 1950 it took 23 minutes to earn enough money to buy a pint of beer, and $6\frac{1}{2}$ hours for a bottle of whisky. By 1976 this had fallen to 12 minutes and 2 hours respectively.

## The unit of alcohol

All the recent work on alcohol and its abuse uses the idea of the unit of alcoholic drink. One unit contains between 8 and 10 g of pure alcohol. This amount is contained in half a pint of beer or lager, one glass of wine or a pub measure of spirits. A bottle of spirits is 40 units and a bottle of wine 7 units. A can of beer is $1\frac{1}{2}$ units. Extra-strength beers or fortified wines have more alcohol.

Home measures are generally about twice pub measures.

## What are the dangers of alcohol overuse?

The vast majority of adults in this country drink some alcohol, with only 6% of men and 11% of women reporting themselves as complete abstainers.[1] Thus non-drinkers do not constitute a representative sample of the general population.

A few people drink alcohol to considerable excess. Six per cent of men drink over 50 units a week and 1% of women drink over 36 units a week.[1] These people are at clear risk of damage.

The vast majority of people drink at a level between these extremes. Each of them has only a slight risk of drink damage. However, the number of people who fall in this group is so large that the cumulative total damage caused is greater than that suffered by the much smaller numbers of very heavy drinkers.

### Death from alcohol-induced illness

There are estimated to be 28 000 excess deaths per year in the UK because of alcohol.[3] There is evidence of a U-shaped relationship between an individual's alcohol consumption and the risk of death. The risks of accidents, stroke and liver disease are apparent at drinking levels of over 21 units a week.

People who consume less than 7 units a week have slightly higher mortality rates than the lowest, even when allowing for the potential confounding factor that people who are already ill will tend to drink less. Overall, the lowest mortality is achieved by drinking between 7 and 21 units a week.[4]

### Heart disease

The increase in heart disease seen in heavy drinkers does not become apparent until consumption levels are over 40 units a week. Levels below 7 units a week are associated with a slightly increased risk of heart disease.[4]

Some types of alcoholic drink may be safer than others. This might explain the so-called French paradox, which is that, though alcohol consumption in France is high by international standards, none the less the heart attack rate is low. From this it is speculated that red wine in particular may have protective properties. Red wine contains many things as well as alcohol, and it may be the antioxidants and trace elements which have a beneficial effect on blood coagulability.[5]

## Hypertension

In between 10 and 30% of cases of hypertension, alcohol is the principal or sole cause. This effect is reversible on abstinence.[6]

## Road accidents

Alcohol is responsible for about 1000 road traffic accident deaths per year, or 20% of the total. Up to 50% of persons killed in road traffic accidents are over the legal alcohol driving limit. Between 10 p.m. and 4 a.m. on Friday and Saturday nights, two-thirds of drivers and motorbike riders have alcohol levels above the legal limit. Drinking is involved in 45% of road accidents with young people.[7]

## Other accidents

Alcohol is involved in 50% of murders, 20% of child abuse, 65% of suicides, 20% of drownings, 35% of domestic accidents and 60% of serious head injuries.[8]

Some 20% of people admitted to hospitals have problems with alcohol abuse.[9] Fourteen per cent of attendances at accident and emergency departments are due to alcohol. Between 8 p.m. and midnight the figure is 24% and between midnight and 6 a.m. it is 46%.[10]

## Drinking and pregnancy[2]

The risk of spontaneous abortion is increased in women who drink alcohol when pregnant.

### Fetal alcohol syndrome
This affects 1–2 per 1000 live births, and may be seen when the mother has drunk more than 70 units a week during pregnancy.
Features are:

- Characteristic facies:
  Microcephaly.

Short palpebral fissure.
Flattened maxillary area.
Microphthalmia.
Flat upper lip.
Anteverted nostrils.
- Pre- or postnatal growth retardation.
- Central nervous system involvement.

*Fetal alcohol effects*
These are seen in 2–3 per 1000 live births, and may be brought about by maternal drinking over 35 units a week during pregnancy.
Features are:

- Cerebral abnormality – small head.
- Mental retardation.
- Neonatal jitteriness.
- Hyperactivity.
- Speech and learning delay.
- Abnormalities of central nervous system, limbs, heart, liver.
- Immunological deficiency and thus more infections.

Up to 8% of all mental retardation may be attributable to alcohol ingestion.
A pregnant woman who drinks 10 units a week approximately doubles the risk of a small-for-dates baby. There is probably no completely safe level of drinking during pregnancy, but failing complete abstinence, it is advisable to limit intake to 2 units on any given occasion.

## How much does it cost?

In 1983 it was estimated that road accidents directly attributable to the overuse of alcohol cost the country £178m a year.[7]
In 1989, sickness absence associated with alcohol consumption cost £779m in the UK, and the costs to the National Health Service were estimated at £120m.[3]

## What is safe drinking?

Finding the safe limit for alcohol consumption has proved difficult, but over the years there has been a downwards trend in what is considered safe. Current orthodoxy is that for men, over 21 units a week is harmful, and for women 14 units.[9] During 1994 it was announced, however, that the Department of Health was reconsidering its guidance as a result of the increasing weight of evidence that a moderate alcohol consumption confers some protection from illness.

Medical harm is possible when drinking over 50 units a week, and probable in those drinking more than 90 units.

## How much do people drink?

Twenty-seven per cent of men in the UK drink more than 21 units a week, and 7% drink more than 50 units. Thirteen per cent of women in the UK drink more than 14 units per week, and 2% drink more than 36 units.[3]

In an average GP list of 2000, there will be 40 physically dependent drinkers (of whom half will be known), 160 problem drinkers, 960 healthy drinkers and 80 non-drinkers.[10]

Five to 12 per cent of men and 1–2% of women over 65 are problem drinkers.[11] The problems caused are made worse by frailty, coexisting illnesses and by medication.

Thirty per cent of 13 year olds and 50% of 15 year olds are drinking alcohol at least once a week.[12]

Some occupational groups have a higher than average chance of death from cirrhosis of the liver. The standardized mortality ratio for cirrhosis among publicans is 1576, for doctors is 311, and for farmers is under 50.[1]

## What can be done?

Two strategies have been proposed for reducing alcohol damage: the high-risk approach and the population approach.

### High-risk approach

The small group of heavy drinkers are targeted for treatment.

### Population approach

The aim is to reduce average alcohol consumption, as most alcohol damage is seen in the large numbers of people who drink only slightly more than is good for them.

In fact the two approaches are not conflicting. The number of alcohol-damaged people in a community is closely related to the average alcohol consumption of that community. A general reduction in consumption will hence reduce the numbers of problem drinkers. The heavier drinkers reduce their consumption as well as the lighter drinkers.[13]

The *Health of the Nation*[14] has set a target of reducing the number of men consuming over 21 units of alcohol per week from 28 to 18%, and the proportion of women consuming more than 14 units of alcohol per week from 11 to 7% by the year 2001.

The Department of Health estimates that a 1% increase in the price of alcohol leads to a 1% reduction in consumption.[3] Each year £17 000m is spent in this country on alcoholic drinks, and a large part of this goes to the exchequer.[10] Alcohol is big business, with significant revenue implications for government. This may explain the lukewarm attitude of successive governments towards controlling alcohol consumption through fiscal means.

# How to recognize a problem drinker

## Suspicious presentations

Some clinical presentations should make the GP suspect that alcohol consumption is causing damage.[9]

*Physical*
- Gastrointestinal symptoms, e.g. vomiting, diarrhoea, Monday morning gastritis.
- Trauma, e.g. injuries, accidents, burns.
- Fractures, especially rib fractures.
- Collapse, fits, faints.
- Withdrawal symptoms, e.g. shakes, night sweats.
- Presenting at the surgery smelling of alcohol.
- Obesity, especially in young males.
- Hypertension.
- Jaundice.

*Psychological*
- Anxiety symptoms.
- Depression.
- Sexual problems.
- Drug abuse, especially benzodiazepines.
- Inappropriate behaviour in surgery.

*Familial*
- Psychological problems in spouse.
- Psychological problems in children.
- Spouse battering.
- Child abuse.

*Social*
- Financial problems, debt.
- Legal problems, criminal, civil, driving offences.
- Work problems, absenteeism, frequent job change, dismissal.

## Ask the patient

The GP will wish to establish how much alcohol the patient is consuming without causing offence. The GP contract requires a record to be made of patients' admitted alcohol consumption. The more this happens, the more people become accustomed to the idea of being asked, and so the less offence it will cause.

A question about alcohol can be asked as part of a general enquiry about lifestyle, including diet, smoking and exercise habits. From a diagnostic standpoint, the clinician cannot afford to ignore the effects of habits on health. If the patient appears to be taking offence, it can be pointed out that all avenues need to be explored so that the problem can be identified and treated properly. A reluctance by the patient to divulge information about drinking can in itself indicate that there may be a problem, of which the patient is already partly aware.

Patients often underestimate the amount they drink. There are a number of possible reasons for this:

- It is not moral to drink to excess. The memory of the temperance leagues is still abroad.
- Patients may make genuine errors in estimating the amount they have consumed.
- Patients may not wish their symptoms to be dismissed as due to alcohol for fear of a serious pathology being missed.

A drinking history can be taken by reference to the last 7 days. Many problem drinkers will tell you that the last week has been unusual in some respect, leading to more than average consumption.[9]

## The drink diary

The history can be reinforced by inviting the patient to fill in a drink diary. A number of published examples are available, or the patient can construct his or her own.

On each day get the patient to record:

- How much was drunk.
- What were the circumstances of the drinking?
- How he or she felt before and after the drinking.
- What, if any, were the consequences of the drinking?

Over the course of 2 weeks it will be possible to get an accurate assessment of the amount drunk, and also gain some insight into why the drinking behaviour is occurring.

### CAGE questionnaire[15]

The use of questionnaires is known to increase the GP detection rate of problem drinkers.[3] The CAGE form has been used since 1974.

The questions are:

1. Have you ever felt you should *C*ut down on your drinking?
2. Have people ever *A*nnoyed you by criticizing your drinking?
3. Have you ever felt *G*uilty about your drinking?
4. Have you ever had a drink first thing in the morning to steady your nerves or to get rid of a hangover (*E*ye-opener)?

If two or more questions are answered in the affirmative, then there is an 80–90% chance that a drinking problem exists.[9]

## What to do with the results – the at-risk patient

Patients will be detected who show no signs of alcohol damage, but who are drinking at a level which may cause problems in future. This group should be encouraged to reduce their drinking to a safe level.

General advice or even a leaflet may help. A number of people find they are drinking more than they mean to, and the following tips will help prevent this:[9]

- Take smaller sips.
- Occupy yourself – play a game, or talk, or eat.
- Change the drink – this breaks old habits.
- Drink for the taste.
- Imitate the slow drinker.

- Put the glass down between sips.
- Dilute spirits.
- Try and avoid rounds, or miss yourself out on your round.
- Eat first. The alcohol absorption is slowed.
- Take days off drinking altogether.
- Start later.
- Learn to refuse drinks. This may take practice.


## How to help the physically dependent patient

A few patients will be heavily dependent and detoxification may be necessary. Patients who get withdrawal symptoms are physically dependent, and are best dealt with by psychiatrists. The chance of a withdrawal syndrome is greatest with heavier drinkers, but the amount consumed is not the only consideration when assessing the likelihood of a withdrawal reaction.[16]

Withdrawal symptoms begin after 3–6 hours without drinking, and last 5–7 days or occasionally longer.

Up until 12 hours the early symptoms are of tremor, sweating, anorexia, nausea, insomnia and anxiety.

Between 10 and 60 hours there is a risk of withdrawal seizures. These are generalized and may precede or accompany delirium tremens.

After 72 hours delirium tremens may occur with severe tremor, confusion, disorientation, agitation, visual and auditory hallucinations and paranoid ideation. Around 5% of patients withdrawing from alcohol develop delirium tremens, and 10% of these die.[15]

Most patients needing detoxification will require admission to hospital.

Occasionally, in the following cases, it may be possible to detoxify a patient at home:

Patient otherwise healthy.
Good family support.
Symptoms of dependence mild.
Patient says he or she will cooperate with treatment.

Withdrawal symptoms can be relieved using a benzodiazepine, usually chlordiazepoxide at a dose of 10–15 mg three or four times a day, with a maximum of 40 mg four times a day. The dose is tailed off to zero over 7–10 days. Chlormethiazole is now considered safe for hospital practice only because of the risks of dependence and respiratory depression.[16]

# How to help the alcohol-damaged patient

The presence of alcohol damage usually comes to light in one of four ways, in order of frequency:

- A physical or emotional crisis has arisen because of drinking.
- A spouse or other family member or a friend attends to tell you of his or her suspicions.
- The patient presents with a problem which may be related to drinking.
- Evidence of alcohol damage and excess consumption is detected during routine screening.

It is important to take notice of what concerned carers may tell you, as their assessment will usually be more accurate than the story you obtain from the patient. In addition, it is they who have to tolerate the results of the drinking, and so they deserve consideration. Carers are also a crucial part of attempts at treatment.

This said, a treatment cannot be imposed on the patient. The patient must be sufficiently aware that the drinking is causing or at least aggravating a problem to present for help. Such awareness may not be permanent, so that one day he or she will admit that drink is a problem, and the next he or she may be equally convinced that the only reason he or she drinks is because the world is so awful.

A psychiatric illness will commonly coexist with the heavy drinking, and it is often difficult to sort out whether the psychiatric problem or the drink problem is the primary cause of the patient's symptoms.

# How to convince a patient that he or she is drinking too much

Patients may wish to reduce their drinking for a variety of reasons. The reduction of illness may be of prime importance to the doctor, but patients are just as likely to be concerned about the cost and the weight gain resulting from their drinking.

### Drinking diary

This may convince the partially aware of how much they are drinking.

## Drinking comparison

This will show the patient where he or she falls in comparison to the general population.[9]

*Men*
Nil 6%
Occasional 18%
1–5 units 20%
6–10 units 13%
11–20 units 17%
21–35 units 13%
36–50 units 8%
Over 50 units 6%

*Women*
Nil 11%
Occasional 31%
1–5 units 34%
6–10 units 10%
11–20 units 10%
21–35 units 2%
Over 35 units 1%

## Firm advice

Sometimes the doctor can use sapiential and moral authority to motivate the patient. In transactional analysis terms this is the parent doctor addressing the child patient.

## Blood tests

$\gamma$-Glutamyl transferase (GGT) and full blood count (FBC) may help confirm that drinking is at a level where demonstrable changes are occurring. Mean corpuscular volume (MCV) is raised in 45–50% of alcohol-dependent patients (compared with 1–2% of the normal population). A raised GGT and MCV will identify 90% of alcohol-dependents.[17]

## Profit and loss balance

Drinkers usually have reasons for drinking, and so see advantages as well as disadvantages from continued heavy drinking. The patient can be helped to draw up a personal list of reasons for continuing to drink heavily, and for reducing. This list can be used later to focus on the patient's own reasons for wanting to reduce drinking.

## Advice

When trying to help a patient, the advice offered needs to be personalized, specific and concrete. Use the information gathered to tailor a care package for that individual.

## Motivational interviewing[18]

This technique was developed to help alcohol-dependent patients become motivated to cut down their consumption. It is a method of attitude alteration (moving people from contemplation to action) based on two observations:

- If one person develops one viewpoint, the other person will tend to argue the opposite view.
- If a person says something often enough, he or she will come to believe it.

To use this effect, it is important not to present the issue of alcohol consumption in a threatening way. Otherwise, the patient will take the opposite view, and will come to believe more and more that alcohol is not the problem. It is also important to keep the drinking on the agenda. Information from the 'profit and loss account' can be particularly useful.

The following are suggested:

- Work with the patient's own framework. Keep the emphasis on the patient's own reasons for wanting to cut consumption. You don't have to think of yourself as an alcoholic to want to reduce your drinking.
- Encourage the patient to emphasize his or her own role in drinking. It's no good constantly blaming external factors.
- Discussing the advantages and disadvantages of drinking can be a powerful motivation. It is important, however, not to make assumptions. The patient may not want to stay alive, or to save his or her marriage.
- Empathize with the wish to change drinking habits, but also with the difficulties of doing this.
- Pick out patient statements which demonstrate the patient's own reasons for wanting to cut down.
- Discuss factual issues, for example the results of blood tests.

- Use cognitive dissonance to challenge statements without causing offence. An example would be: 'You say on one hand that you drink because you are in debt, but you also say the drinking is costing you a lot of money. I don't understand.'

## Staying stopped

The patient's progress should be reviewed at intervals. Success should be praised and a further attempt encouraged if there has been a failure. Motivation to stop may not always be present. If there has been a relapse, start again. It often takes several goes before success is achieved.

- Look for what has triggered any relapse. Avoiding the trigger may help future attempts.
- Keep contact with other family members and any other health workers who have been involved. It is best if everybody concerned is saying the same things. A united front is required.
- Continue to monitor input, and reinforce with repeated blood tests if needed. Enquire about other problems, e.g. impotence, work problems, etc.

## Cravings

As alcohol is a tranquillizer, its withdrawal may be associated with anxiety symptoms. Anxiety and the fear of anxiety may be equally troublesome.

Anxiety-lowering techniques may help, such as sequential muscle contraction or breathing exercises. More complex devices such as meditation or relaxation tapes may be useful.

## Will it work?

A review of available evidence in 1993[3] concluded that brief intervention by GPs was effective and should reduce alcohol consumption by up to 20% in people with a high consumption. However, it is not clear how such a change would translate into changes in health status.

It is estimated that such intervention would cost about £20 per patient in 1993 prices, and that non-specialist intervention is just as likely to succeed as specialist care.

It should be noted that brief intervention in this context is rather more than just the normal GP consultation. In the trials showing benefit, the GPs had special training and presumably a special interest. The interviews were longer than average, and needed repeating up to four times. Severely affected drinkers were excluded from the surveys. Also, only just over half the patients identified as being at risk turned up for treatment.

## Problem situations[9]

### Suicide threats

The suicide rate is high in alcohol abusers, and drunkenness may lower the threshold for an impetuous act. An assessment must be made of suicide risk, and if this is significant then admission may be needed. The Mental Health Act can be used if the patient is at risk of self-harm.

### Violence

Violence is common, and the police may need to be involved. Consider child abuse procedures if appropriate. Delusional jealousy among husbands is particularly troublesome.

### Drunk in surgery

Once may be tolerated, but it is impossible to do useful work with someone who is drunk.

## Which patients need referral?

Some patients will need inpatient care because they need detoxi-fication, because they require treatment for an alcohol-induced illness or because their psychological symptoms are so severe that they are a danger to themselves or others. The patient who is not acutely unwell may benefit from a planned admission to withdraw the alcohol.

Out-patient referral will be appropriate for those patients who are not responding to community treatment or who have complicating coexisting psychiatric or physical problems. Where a physical illness is causing concern it will be necessary to take advice from the medical team rather than the psychiatrists.

Other members of the primary health care team can be involved. The key workers here are the community psychiatric nurses. In some areas there may be a community alcohol team who can be referred to. In addition, most alcohol-dependent patients would benefit from contact with one of the self-help organizations involved in alcohol work.

Referral may be considered if:

- There is no progress with treatment.
- There are serious medical complications, e.g. cirrhosis.
- There are severe withdrawal symptoms, especially if there have been fits or delirium tremens.
- Home support is poor.
- There are complicating psychological or family factors.
- Treatment with disulfiram is being considered. There has been a resurgence of interest in this drug,[19] but its use should be restricted to problem cases under specialist care.

## Self-help groups

### Alcoholics anonymous

Alcoholics anonymous is a voluntary fellowship of alcoholics who help each other through group meetings and a 12-step programme to recovery. There are about 2300 groups around the country. There is a slightly religious attitude to the problem which some people are unable to tolerate.

PO Box 1, Stonebow House, Stonebow, York YO1 2NJ. 01904 644026.

### Al-Anon

Al-Anon is a self-help group for the family and friends of problem drinkers. There are over 1000 local groups. Alateen is a subsection for teenagers whose lives are being affected by somebody else's drinking.

61 Great Dover Street, London SE1 4YF.
0171 430 0888.

### Councils on alcoholism

These provide voluntary counselling to drinkers and families, and are present in the larger population centres.

# References

1. *Alcohol – A Balanced View. Report from General Practice no. 24*. London: Royal College of General Practitioners 1986
2. *Alcohol and Child Development*. BMA symposium, 30th November 1983
3. *Effective Health Care. Brief Interventions and Alcohol Use*. Nuffield Institute for Health, University of Leeds; Centre for Health Economics, University of York; Research Unit, Royal College of Physicians 1993
4. Kemm J. Alcohol and heart disease: the implications of the U-shaped curve. *Br Med J* 1993: **307**: 1373–4
5. *Alcohol and Cardiovascular Diseases. Factfile*. British Heart Foundation. 1993
6. Sanders JB. Alcohol: an important cause of hypertension. *Br Med J* 1987; **294**: 1045–6
7. Thomson AD (ed) *Licence to Kill? Alcoholism no 3*. London: Medical Council on Alcoholism 1987
8. *The Guardian* 23 May 1992
9. *Hazardous Drinking*. London: Medical Council on Alcoholism 1987
10. Anderson P. Alcohol epidemiology. *The Practitioner* 1991; **235**: 594
11. Dunne FJ. Misuse of alcohol or drugs by elderly people. *Br Med J* 1994; **308**: 608–9
12. Hoskins T. Alcohol abuse in children. *Maternal and Child Health* 1989; **14**(7): 194–6
13. Dillner L. Alcohol abuse. *Br Med J* 1991; **302**: 859–60
14. Secretary of State for Health. *The Health of the Nation: A Strategy for Health in England*. London: HMSO 1992
15. Mayfield D, McLeod G & Hall P. The CAGE questionnaire. *Am J Psychiatry* 1974; **131**: 1121–3
16. Alcohol problems in the general hospital. *Drug Ther Bull* 1991; **29**: 18
17. Bloor RN. Social drinker? Detecting and assessing alcohol problems. *Update* 1993; 24–30
18. Miller WR. Motivational interviewing with problem drinkers. *Behav Psychother* 1983; **11**: 147–72
19. Heather N. Disulfiram treatment for alcoholism. *Br Med J* 1989; **299**: 471–2

# 10

# Managing psychiatric emergencies

## Aims

The trainee should:

- Be able to recognize the clinical syndromes which may present acutely.
- Be able to assess the risks posed by a given clinical situation and respond accordingly.
- Have knowledge of the relevant provisions of the Mental Health Act 1983.

## Introduction

With the move towards community management of more severely psychiatrically ill patients, GPs can expect an increased workload from emergency situations in future.

The tolerance of difficult behaviour is related to the circumstances. Behaviour tolerable in the day may not be tolerated in the night. Changes in carers may alter the crisis threshold in a particular case. Difficult behaviour at unsocial times is more likely to precipitate a crisis and require GP intervention.

A crisis and hence an emergency visit request will usually result from:[1]

- Violence or threats of violence.
- Suicidal or self-harm behaviour.
- Behaviour which is socially inappropriate in the circumstances – weeping, shouting, wandering outside in the middle of the night.

Family, friends and neighbours are more likely to request the visit than is the patient. The request for an urgent visit is often used as an index of concern for the patient rather than because of a sudden worsening of symptoms.

A visit from a doctor, or indeed the police or a priest, can in itself have a calming effect, especially with acute anxiety problems.

Treatment of a psychiatric emergency should concentrate on how to get over the next 24–48 hours.[1] It is nearly impossible to solve a chronic problem in the middle of the night. Admission to hospital may be the only way to 'buy time' to allow the crisis to settle.

In patients under 60, most emergency psychiatric calls are for acute anxiety or alcohol/drug intoxication. In patients over 60, the majority are for dementia and toxic confusional states.

## An overview of psychiatric emergencies

When dealing with an acutely disturbed patient and carers, it is easy to get sucked into the thought disorder with the patient so that you find yourself debating and sometimes arguing the nature of reality. This is unhelpful. It is necessary to take one step back and assess the behaviour objectively, while looking for symptom patterns in order to make the diagnosis. The more patterns you are familiar with, the more chance there is of making an accurate assessment.

This clinical attitude runs counter to the normal GP–patient interface where empathy is used to elicit useful information. Under usual circumstances, presenting complaints are taken at face value and dealt with within the patient's own understanding. When the patient presents with difficult behaviour, however, it may not be possible to agree with the patient what the problem is.

On the other hand, some difficult behaviour may be understandable in the light of the circumstances, or in the context of the relationships which the patient has with those around and with the practitioner. The GP's assessment should be objective and based on evidence, as with all problem situations. The practitioner who too readily assumes that difficult behaviour is due to a mental illness or a personality disorder in reality displays a lack of coping and consultation skills.

The prime relationship which carers and family members have with the patient is one of sympathy. Carers will hence have particular difficulty seeing unusual behaviour as part of an illness pattern. The least able people to cope with a confused patient are those who know them best. Unfortunately, these are the same familiar group in whose care the patient is likely to be least disturbed and most compliant.

## Mania and hypomania

The difference between hypomania and mania is only of degree, with mania being the more exaggerated variety.

Isolated mania is uncommon and most episodes arise in the context of a bipolar affective disorder. In the early stages the change in behaviour is usually put down to high spirits and as such is not only acceptable but a positive social asset. It then becomes apparent that the behaviour is getting out of hand, with high energy and distractability, constant physical and mental activity and increased appetites. The tendency to spend money can have particularly unfortunate longer-term consequences. Patients will also make excessive demands on those around them to keep up with the rush of energy and ideas.

The problem is usually first brought to light by the exhausted spouse. There may have been a gradual worsening of symptoms so that the situation is often quite far advanced before being brought to medical attention. The GP is usually in a better position to detect the disorder because being confronted with florid manic behaviour creates more impact than does witnessing the gradual worsening of the situation.

Once there has been one episode of mania, any further episodes are easier for the family to identify. Mania usually arises in patients already known to be prone to the problem, and so new cases are rare.

Common features of mania include mood elevation, irritability and hostility, pressure of talk, flight of ideas and impairment of insight. Delusions, usually grandiose, are present, with increased sexual drive and hallucinations. Motor overactivity leading to exhaustion and dehydration may occur.

## Functional disorders

These are secondary to a psychiatric disorder. Their main difference from the organic psychoses is that the conscious level is not impaired.

### Schizophrenia

This may present as an acute psychotic episode, especially in the younger patient. A change in personality may be noticed by the family in the recent past. In making the diagnosis, positive features (Schneider's first-rank symptoms) may include:[2]

- Hallucinations, typically auditory.
- Thought insertion.
- Thought withdrawal.
- Thought broadcasting.

- Passivity.
- Primary delusions, often paranoid.

Negative features include:

- Lack of insight.
- Loss of interest or enjoyment.
- Flat, blunted affect. There may seem to be a 'pane of glass' between you and the patient so that communication is distorted.
- Poor speech.
- Loss of initiative and drive.
- Social withdrawal and isolation.

### Depression

Depressed people are often highly dependent and irritating company, with their poor self-esteem, gloomy foreboding about the future and social withdrawal. They are more likely to harm themselves than others, but violent behaviour may occur. In particular, mothers suffering postnatal depression may harm their babies.

### Acute anxiety

Acute episodes may be seen as new episodes, or against a background of anxiety disorder. Symptoms often come on for an identifiable reason – a shock, bad news or an argument. Somatic symptoms such as sweats, palpitations, tingling, crushing chest pain and dyspnoea may predominate. There may be overt panic or hyperventilation.

There are usually no psychotic features, but there is often evidence of a precipitant, and a history of similar previous events.

### Developmental disorder

Impulsivity and a poor capacity to adapt to changing situations by people with a mental handicap can lead to inappropriate social behaviour. Other social disadvantages tend to complicate the picture.

## Organic psychosis

Some people are particularly susceptible to toxic confusional states. If brain reserves are low, small degrees of insult may lead to significant reaction. As brain failure is much more common in the elderly population, demography indicates that we will all be seeing a lot more of this in future.

A prime feature of this group is clouding of consciousness, and this is the chief way of distinguishing the organic from the functional disorders.

## Toxic confusion

*Signs and symptoms of toxic confusion*
1. Reduced conscious awareness:

   - Failure to understand instructions.
   - Disorientation in time and space.
   - Reluctance to cooperate.
   - Delusions of persecution.
   - Fluctuations in conscious level.

2. Restlessness. Plucking at bed covers.
3. Irritability.
4. Sleep pattern reversal. Awake at night, asleep in the day.
5. Hallucinations, particularly visual.
6. Dysphasia.
7. Perseveration and disconnected thinking.
8. Anxiety.

## What can cause toxic confusion?

Any extra stress may cause an acute confusion in the predisposed. All infections can bring about such stress, but some sites of infection are common precipitants. Organ failure can produce similar reactions.

- Respiratory failure.
- Infection, especially pneumonia in the elderly, but don't forget urinary tract infection.
- Intoxication – often alcohol, but may be drugs, prescribed or otherwise.
- Drug withdrawal; Delirium tremens.
- Alcohol withdrawal; Wernicke's encephalopathy.
- Constipation.

If an underlying organic disorder is found, then treatment is directed towards this as well as towards the confusion. The existence of toxic confusion means that there is probably reduced function in many organic systems, and so the side-effects of any treatments may be exaggerated, and dosages of medication used should have regard to the likely efficiency of the patient's elimination systems such as renal and hepatic function.

## Brain failure: dementia

As well as making the sufferer more likely to get delirium, the dementias by themselves can result in challenging behaviour. The same person will often have failure of other sensory modes such as vision or proprioception. Falls are more likely, so the possibility of intracranial bleed must be borne in mind.

The patient is usually elderly. There will have been a gradual deterioration in social, intellectual and often physical functioning. The situation will have been held in control until a change in circumstances has occurred. This change may be a deterioration in the condition or a supervening illness which has increased the patients' dependence on their carers. Alternatively there may have been a change for the carer, such as illness or an imminent holiday.

Entering a situation where the caring structure is breaking down, it is not uncommon to feel resentful of the carers for withdrawing their support and so generating the crisis. It is worth bearing in mind that the carers have often been struggling against major problems for years. Many of them will have given up work for their unpaid caring role, or may well be elderly or ill themselves. Whether the change in the carers is their inability or unwillingness to carry on makes little objective difference.

When you hear phrases like 'I'm ill myself, you know' you can be sure the carers are near to giving up. Once the decision has been made to get the doctor in, there will be a tendency to play up the problems to support their decision. Admission is often needed to buy some time for the carers and stabilize the patient's clinical situation. After a break, carers will often be prepared to resume some caring activity.

Day care, respite care, phased admissions or help bought in through the use of the Attendance Allowance can help to keep the patient and carers going a bit longer. Good lighting, familiar surroundings and an environment free from accident hazards help with confidence for all concerned.

## Is the patient really ill?

Personality disorder is often used as a term of medical abuse, and as such is singularly unhelpful.[3] However, some people seem unable to resist their impulses, and need their wishes gratifying instantly. This often makes their interactions with health professionals rather abrasive. Unfortunately, an impulsive personality is a risk factor for suicide, so the natural tendency to retaliate must be tempered by professional considerations. The making of contracts and the setting down of ground rules is often effective.

A psychosocial crisis may give rise to requests for medical attention. Arguments between partners can cause individual distress, and the summoning of the doctor can be used to prove a point, or settle an argument. This may lead to the disconcerting experience of urgently attending a call to find the 'patient' sound asleep.

Violent behaviour is becoming more common, both in psychiatric cases, and in the normal day-to-day work of the GP. In 1992, the General Medical Services Committee of the British Medical Association produced their own guidance for avoiding and dealing with violent behaviour.[13]

Basically, giving in seems to be the best way of avoiding incidents when faced with a potentially violent patient.[4] Keeping door-side of the patient ensures a line of retreat, and some advocate sitting on the chair with the back in front to serve as a barrier if necessary.

Sections 4 and 5 of the 1986 Public Order Act make it an offence to use threatening behaviour in other than a dwelling place, but this legislation provides no protection during a home visit. The Offences Against the Person Act can be used after an actual assault: this is the same Act that can cause problems if you examine a patient without his or her permission.

From 1 April 1994, there has been a change in the GP contract which allows GPs to remove from their list with immediate effect any patient who has been violent or who has behaved in a way to cause the GP to be afraid that violence towards the GP may occur. The GP still retains a duty to provide medical care in an emergency, but if this occurs then it is advised that there be a police presence during the consultation. The GP has no duty to render non-emergency care.

As well as removing the patient from the list, the GP can take out an injunction to stop the patient coming to the surgery. The patient is not deprived of medical services since on re-registration elsewhere, services can be obtained straight away.

## What to do when called to an acute psychiatric emergency

Before attending a psychiatric emergency, it is important to gather as much background information as possible. At first this can be got from the request call and the records: this is an occasion when access to the past medical notes is particularly useful.

Many of the patients you are called to see in these circumstances will be well known to the practice and to the psychiatric services. There may have been previous urgent requests for attention, and the outcome of these will give a good idea of how the present crisis will need to be handled.

Calls are seldom so urgent that you have to drop everything to attend, but neither should the delay be too long. It is often possible over the phone to buy some time. A brief delay before attending can help clarify the clinical situation, and also gives you a chance to prepare yourself for what will be a longer than average consultation.

## Making a psychological assessment

At attendance, the history from the relatives is most important. The premorbid personality of the patient and the sequence of events can be elicited, as can the particular reason why the visit request has been made now. A calm and systematic approach is mandatory.

Well-prepared with information from the carers, during the consultation with the patient it is possible to concentrate on the symptoms which would confirm the diagnosis suggested by the carers' history. In addition the particular pieces of behaviour which have caused the crisis can be specifically enquired about.

Making a definitive diagnosis during a crisis is not necessary, and neither is it usually possible. If the Mental Health Act might have to be used it is important to establish that a psychiatric illness exists. A decision about whether or not a section of the Mental Health Act should be invoked depends on the following:

- Is the patient a risk to him or herself or others?
- Is treatment required and will the patient cooperate with such treatment?

## Is the patient a risk to him/herself? Assessing suicidal risk

In 1990 there were 4485 official suicides in the UK, and probably at least as many again go unrecognized (for instance, suicide is a venial sin for Roman Catholics). There has been a 50% increase in suicide in males under 25 in the last 10 years, so it is now the commonest single cause of death in this age group[5]

*Health of the Nation* targets are to reduce the suicide rate by 15% in the general population, and by 33% in the severely mentally ill.[6]

*Who might kill themselves?*
Patients who have the following characteristics are more at risk of committing suicide:[7]

- Current or former psychiatric patients (inpatient or outpatient): 10 times risk.
- Within 4 weeks of discharge from a psychiatric hospital: men 200 times risk, women 100 times risk.
- History of parasuicide: 10–30 times risk, and there is also a 60-fold increase in the risk of death by 'natural causes'.[8]
- Alcohol abusers: 20 times risk.
- Drug misusers: 20 times risk.
- Acquired immune deficiency syndrome (AIDS) sufferers: 36 times risk.
- Doctors, farmers, unemployed: 2 times risk.
- Young Asian women: 2.7 times risk.
- Samaritan clients: 20 times risk. Except in some groups, in particular young white women, the existence of a Samaritan service in an area does not seem to have any effect on the rate of suicide in that area.[7]

And also in women:[9]

- Loss of mother by death or separation before age 12.
- Three or more children under 5.
- Lack of either a close caring relationship or a job.

*Can suicide be prevented?*
Forty per cent of patients who complete suicide will have seen their GP in the preceding month, and 20% within the preceding week.[7] Unfortunately, the younger patients are less likely to have had contact with their GP. Of patients who commit suicide, 30% are known to the psychiatric services. Most in retrospect have a recognizable psychiatric disorder – usually, but not always, depression.

It is sensible to ask the patient about suicidal thoughts and plans. Asking never 'gives them ideas': most depressed people have at least wondered what it would be like to be dead, and are often relieved to share their feelings. Feelings of wanting to 'get away from it all' are pretty normal.

If the patient is making plans to commit suicide, has feelings of worthlessness, and also falls into one of the at-risk groups, then the risk of suicide is substantial.

### Is the patient a risk to others?

It is very unusual for a patient to be dangerous to others because of a psychiatric disorder. Schizophrenic patients may have paranoid delusions which sometimes cause them to direct aggression towards others. Patients with mania or hypomania may feel that their grandiose schemes are being prevented and this may lead to boisterous frustration or even frank aggression. Patients with personality disorder may be unable to tolerate situations where their whims are not met.

Patients with toxic confusion are usually restless and may have hallucinations which cause aggressive behaviour. Because of the clouding of consciousness, such aggression is not well-directed so the risk of harm is slight.

A patient who is behaving aggressively causes great concern to carers. If violence has occurred, the police should be involved at an early stage, together with an approved social worker, as the two major management options are sectioning or arrest.

In situations where violence is threatened, it may still be possible to make a psychological assessment unless the violence is being threatened towards the GP. None the less it is as well to attend backed-up by a social worker, with the police alerted but keeping a discreet distance while negotiations proceed. If the patient requires hospitalization (rather than arrest), then informal admission is unlikely to be accepted.

### Will the patient co-operate with treatment?

Most patients encountered in emergency situations are only too keen to accept treatment since they feel wretched. This is particularly true for the acute anxieties and the psychosocial crises which form the bulk of the psychiatric emergencies seen.

The depressed will usually agree to treatment unless their symptoms of guilt are so strong that they are reluctant to let anybody else help them.

The patient with hallucinations and delusions is less likely to go along with treatment. None the less, most schizophrenics are not particularly happy people and may well go along with a negotiated plan to relieve them. Having once agreed to treatment, however, this does not mean that they will not change their mind.

Patients with mania will often have little or no insight into their illness. They feel fine; it's the rest of the world that's suffering. Compulsory admission is often required.

The patient with toxic confusion is not usually in a position to give or withhold consent to treat. They will usually require medical rather than primarily psychiatric care.

## Is any physical examination useful?

When seeing the patient, for functional problems no physical examination is needed.

For possible organic problems:

- Take the temperature for pyrexia.
- Listen to the heart and lungs for signs of heart failure and infection.
- Check the abdomen for signs of abdominal pathology and constipation.
- Test the urine for glucose.

Other investigations may be indicated by the history.

## What sort of medication may help?

When considering medication for the acutely disturbed it does not much matter what the underlying problem is. What does matter is the age and general medical condition of the patient.

Medication is preferably given orally, when liquid forms can be particularly useful. Alternatively, they can be given rectally (although not the usual British tradition) or by intramuscular or intravenous injection.

Of the intramuscular preparations, haloperidol is probably the best. It will help in 83% of cases of problem behaviour within 30 minutes.[10] The addition of procyclidine reduces the extrapyramidal problems. The dose is 5–10 mg, using the smaller doses in the old and toxic. An alternative preparation is lorazepam 1–5 mg, but this must be used with caution in patients with respiratory depression.

Of the intravenous options, diazepam in the form of Diazemuls is preferred. It can be given in doses of 5 mg every 15 minutes until the required result is achieved, up to a maximum of 40 mg.

## When is admission needed?

Hospital admission is a tempting way to resolve a psychiatric crisis. The family get the patient off their hands, and are also saved

awkward decisions as to whether the patient's behaviour is pathological or not. The GP gets a potentially disruptive patient out of
his or her hair for a time. It may even be the best way of treating the
patient.

On the other hand, hospital admission disorients the confused,
lowers self-esteem and may reinforce illness behaviour. It is also
expensive.

If admission is on the cards, it is as well to involve the community
psychiatric team at an early stage. The community psychiatric nurse
may be able to make an assessment and negotiate alternatives to
admission with the patient and carers. In many parts of the
country, the hospital psychiatric team will do an urgent home
assessment if an admission is requested, again to see if there is a
better way of handling the crisis.

These assessments are potentially useful as a way of defusing
problem situations, of looking at alternatives, and of assessing what
hospital or outpatient care may have to offer. They can also be used
educationally. On the other hand the GP and carers may be asked
to take on more responsibility than they are prepared for. Also the
GP's position can be undermined if an admission has been
promised which fails to materialize.

Reasons for admission include:[1]

- First psychotic episode.
- Organic psychosis suspected.
- Danger to self or others.
- Unstable patients, poorly supported or poor compliance.

## The Mental Health Act 1983

Since the 16th century there have been legal mechanisms in this
country to deprive of liberty persons whose mental illness makes
them a danger to themselves or others. In 1989/90, there were
17 000 compulsory admissions to psychiatric hospital in the UK, or
around 7% of all psychiatric admissions.[11]

For a patient who refuses informal (non-compulsory) admission,
the Mental Health Act can be used where the following applies:[12]

- The patient is suffering from mental disorder of a nature or
  degree that warrants the detention of the patient in a hospital

  and

- The patient should be so detained in the interests of his or her
  own health or safety or with a view to the protection of others.

A mental disorder can be of four types: mental illness, mental impairment (or mental handicap), severe mental impairment (of degree worse than mental impairment), or psychopathology. The disorder has to be sufficiently severe that the best place for treatment is in hospital. The inclusion of the word health in the phrase 'health or safety' means that the Act also allows for the formal admission of patients who are seriously ill, whether or not they are suicidal or dangerous.[11]

Where two medical recommendations are needed, one should be from a doctor who has been duly accredited as having 'special experience in the diagnosis or treatment of mental disorder' under Section 12 of the same Act (usually a psychiatrist), and the other should preferably have prior knowledge of the patient, usually the patient's GP. Any social workers involved should also be approved, again under the Act, and only a few are so approved.

### Section 2

This lasts up to 28 days, and is for assessment, or assessment and treatment. Application is made by an approved social worker, or by the nearest relative of the patient, who should have seen the patient in the preceding 14 days. Two medical recommendations are needed, and the two doctors should have examined the patient within 5 days of each other.

### Section 3

This lasts up to 6 months and is for treatment. For this section to be used with psychopathic disorder or mental impairment, the admission must be necessary to alleviate or prevent deterioration of the condition. Application is as for section 2, except that if the nearest relative does not agree, then the social worker cannot proceed unless allowed to by a county court. Medical recommendation is also the same, except that the type of mental disorder must be stated.

### Section 4

This is for emergency admission where there isn't time to get a second medical opinion. It lasts 72 hours only. The nearest relative or approved social worker applies, and only one medical recommendation is needed.

This section should only be resorted to in dire emergency.

## Other useful sections

*Section 5 part 2*
This is for someone already in hospital who is there informally, but who becomes sectionable. A single doctor can detain the patient for up to 72 hours to allow a section 2 or 3 to be done.

*Section 5 part 4*
Section 5 part 4 allows a registered mental nurse to detain a sectionable patient up to 6 hours until a doctor can be found.

*Section 136*
Section 136 can be used by a police constable who finds a person who appears to be suffering from a mental disorder in a public place. Under this section the person can be removed to a place of safety (usually a police station or a hospital casualty department) for up to 72 hours for assessment by a doctor or social worker.

*Section 135*
Section 135 allows a police officer to enter a person's home, by force if necessary, with a view to removal to a place of safety.

# How to use the Mental Health Act

Before somebody can be formally admitted, there needs to be somewhere to admit them. A suitable bed has to be found right at the start of the process. Officially the application for formal admission is made to the managers of the admitting unit.

There should be an approved social worker available at all times, but finding one can be difficult. An ordinary social worker will not do. Approved social workers have extra training and are scarce, so they cover a wide catchment.

Forms of application and medical recommendation are available for each different section of the Act. These will guide you through what information is required. They need filling-in completely, and alterations should be initialled.

# When the Mental Health Act cannot be used – common law

There may rarely be circumstances so urgent that immediate restraint or treatment is necessary. When a person poses an immediate danger to him or herself or others, a person acting in good faith may restrain him or her and be protected against accusation of assault by common law.[12] This covers unconscious or overdosed patients.

# References

1. Holmes J. Psychiatric night calls. *The Practitioner* 1990, **234**: 772–5
2. Kenny C. Psychiatry: part 2. *Horizons* 1992; **6**: 515
3. Chiswick D. Mad or bad? *Update* 1993; **46**: 297–300
4. Goss B. Dealing with violent patients. *Med Monitor* 1993; **6**: 14
5. Beecham L. Increase in suicides among the young and elderly. *Br Med J* 1992; **304**: 1344–5
6. Secretary of State for Health. *The Health of the Nation: A Strategy for England.* London: HMSO. 1992
7. Gunnell D & Frankell S. Prevention of suicide: aspirations and evidence. *Br Med J* 1994; **308**: 1227–33
8. Morgan G. Long term risks after attempted suicide. *Br Med J* 1993; **306**: 1626–7
9. Wright A. *Depression: Recognition and Management in General Practice.* London: Royal College of General Practitioners. 1993
10. Management of behavioural emergencies. *Drug Ther Bull* 1991; **29**, August 1991: 62–4
11. Matthews K & Milne S. How and when to apply the Mental Health Act. *The Practitioner* 1994; **238**: 398–404
12. Briscoe M & Harris B. Compulsory detention under the Mental Health Act 1983. *Br Med J* 1987; **294**: 1141–4
13. *Violence against GPs: Time for resolute action.* General Medical Services Committee, London: BMA. 1992

See also Khot and Polmear. *Practical General Practice*, 2nd edn. Butterworth Heinemann: pp. 266–8, 269, 272, 277–8, 338, 341.

# 11

# Cot death

## Aims

The trainee should:

- Know how to manage a baby at high risk of cot death.
- Be able to counsel parents and carers about measures for preventing cot death.
- Be able to detail a management plan to be followed after a cot death.

## How common is cot death?

Cot death is the commonest cause of postneonatal death, accounting for 40% of the deaths seen between the ages of 1 and 12 months.[1] The overall rate is about 2 per 1000 births in the UK, or 1200–1400 each year.[2] The numbers rose gradually from 1950 to 1988, and have fallen steeply since.

Putting this into context, the average GP will have to deal with two cot deaths per professional lifetime and there will be one every 3–4 years in a practice.[3]

## What is a cot death?

Cot death or sudden unexplained death in infancy is a collective term for the situation where a young child is found unexpectedly dead, having been apparently well. There are at least four possible explanations for such an event:[3]

1. Sudden infant death syndrome (SIDS) This is defined as:
   'The sudden death of any infant or young child, which is

unexpected by history, and in which a thorough post-mortem examination fails to demonstrate an adequate cause for death' (Beckwith 1970). The term was coined to explain an observed phenomenon in terms of a legitimate diagnosis which puts no suspicion on parents. However, it has been estimated that up to 10% of SIDS may be infanticide.[4]

The chance of finding a fatal diagnosis depends crucially on the thoroughness of the autopsy. In the UK around 90% of cot deaths proceed to autopsy, but this is not the case in all parts of the world.[4] The Sheffield group report that less than 20% of cot death remains completely unexplained after autopsy and so falls into the true SIDS category.[4]

2. An illness process is present, but of itself this illness would not normally be associated with a fatal outcome.
3. A serious but undetected congenital abnormality is present.
4. An illness process is present which is serious enough to explain the death but which either came on very rapidly or was previously not suspected.

It is estimated that categories 3 and 4 account for no more than 5% of all cot deaths.[3] True SIDS, that is, death for which an autopsy reveals no cause, accounts for around 20% of cot deaths. This leaves by far the biggest category of around 75% in which there has been an abnormally severe reaction to a normally trivial illness which has caused the death.

## Why do some babies react severely to minor illnesses?

A number of theories exist to explain why some babies have such severe reactions to what are usually trivial illnesses. The commonest associated minor ailment is an upper respiratory tract infection (URTI), but such illnesses are almost a permanent feature of babies of this age.

Theories which may explain this reaction include:

1. Upper airways obstruction leading to recurrent episodes of hypoxia.
2. Viraemia following URTI.
3. Hyperthermia due to reduced heat loss because of over-wrapping.
4. Metabolic disorders, especially those resulting in hypoglycaemia.

## Which babies are at risk?

Cot death has generally been studied as a single entity, and not separated into the above four categories. Factors associated with cot death will therefore cover all categories, though doubtless some factors are more relevant to one category than another.

Eighty per cent of cases of cot death occur between the ages of 1 and 6 months, and cases are rare after the first birthday.[3] There is an annual peak in incidence in January, February and March.

Risk factors for cot death can be viewed as avoidable factors and unavoidable factors. Consideration of the avoidable factors forms the basis of the public awareness campaigns. The unavoidable factors provide the basis for the efforts to identify high-risk babies for special attention.

### Unavoidable factors

- Boys are affected slightly more often than girls.
- Low birth weight, prematurity, dysmaturity.
- Twins and higher orders of multiple births are at increased risk.
- Cot death is commoner in cities than in rural areas, and is lower among some ethnic minorities e.g. Afro-Caribbean. The reduced incidence in some groups may be in part due to the practice of small babies sleeping in the same room as the parents.
- Low maternal age.
- Short birth interval.
- Parents unemployed or living in poor housing.
- Maternal infection during pregnancy.
- Mother's failure to attend antenatal and postnatal appointments.
- Maternal drug abuse.
- Some types of delivery, short second stage, lower segment caesarean section, unplanned delivery at home.

### Avoidable factors

- Smoking. Maternal smoking during pregnancy and either parent smoking in the neonatal period increase the chance of a cot death.[5]
- Sleeping in the prone position.
- Not recognizing illness in the baby.
- The baby becoming overheated.
- Bottle-feeding. Breastfeeding has been shown to protect against cot death in the international literature, but has not been shown to be a factor in the UK.

## What advice can be given to parents?

Following studies in Avon and New Zealand, and pressure from the Foundation for the Study of Infant Death (FSID), in 1991 the Department of Health launched its 'Back to Sleep' campaign. By this time there was a wealth of evidence that sleeping position, thermal environment, smoking and recognition of illness were important factors in preventing cot death. Advice leaflets were circulated,[6] and reinforced by a television campaign.

An expert group convened by the Chief Medical Officer reported in November 1993 on the research evidence and made recommendations:[7]

### Sleeping position

Babies who sleep prone are three to eight times more likely to suffer cot death than those who sleep supine. Side sleeping carries an intermediate risk. Babies should be lain supine unless there is a good reason not to, e.g. Pierre Robin syndrome or respiratory problems, but these should be moved to supine as early as practicable.

Side sleeping is all right so long as the lower arm is forwards so that if the baby rolls over it will not end up on its face. It was previously thought that lying babies on their backs would run the risk of them inhaling vomit. This fear is unfounded.[8]

### Smoking

Babies whose parents smoke are two to three times more likely to suffer cot death. Parents should be informed of this risk antenatally and postnatally.

### Temperature control

Overheating carries a risk of cot death of a degree which is substantial but not yet quantified. It is recommended that:

- The room where the baby sleeps should be between 16 and 20°C, i.e. comfortable for a lightly clothed adult. The baby should not be exposed to direct heating, for example, a hot water bottle, when asleep.
- Bedding should not be excessive. Babies need little more bedding than adults. It should be arranged so that the baby cannot slip down under the covers (the head is an important source of heat loss for babies).

- Duvets should not be used for babies under 1 year old. Hats should not be worn in bed beyond the first month unless the room is very cold.

**Breastfeeding**

Breastfeeding is to be encouraged. Internationally there is an association between cot death and bottle-feeding. This has not been found in the UK, but even so breastfeeding is recommended on general health grounds.

**Illness**

Carers who think their baby is unwell should seek medical advice promptly.

This recommendation can be reinforced by the parental use of a scorecard for illness, such as Baby Check.[9] This is a 19-point checklist (12 symptoms and 7 signs) that carers fill in on a daily basis.

In field trials the users of Baby Check felt more secure, and there was an 80–90% agreement between mothers and a specialist nurse as to the state of health of the baby. This should be compared with the 68% agreement which can be expected to be achieved by two clinicians who have seen and examined the same baby.[9]

In the same trials there was found to be no extra demand placed on GP services as a result of the use of Baby Check. Forty-six per cent of mothers found that using the method reduced their anxiety about the child, and only 4% reported their anxiety increased.

## Will advice to parents work?

The incidence of cot death has been falling for some years. After the launch of the Back to Sleep campaign, in the first 9 months of 1992 there were 326 cot deaths, compared to 723 in the first 9 months of 1991 – a reduction of 55%. This compares with reductions of 10–15% in the previous few years, so there has been a marked acceleration of the downward trend following the introduction of the campaign.[8] In addition, it will be noted that the effects of the campaign have been almost immediate.

## How can high-risk babies be identified?

Using the data on cot death risk factors, a number of initiatives have been developed to reduce the chance of cot death by working out an approximate risk for each baby and targeting those at highest risk for special monitoring.

The first large-scale scheme was begun in Sheffield in 1973. Prior to this, Sheffield had consistently had a higher level of cot death than the national average. An initial 2-year pilot scheme showed that increased health visitor and paediatric intervention improved the chances for the high-risk group so identified, and the scheme was extended to the whole city.[3]

All babies resident in Sheffield have assessments done by a health visitor neonatally and at 1 month old. Thirteen potentially adverse social and family factors are enquired about and on the basis of the answers a risk of cot death is worked out.[10] If the score obtained is higher than a threshold of 1 in 160, a special regime of observation is begun with extra health visitor visits and other contacts. GPs are given a black H to stick on to the baby's records.

If a cot death does occur, a meeting is set up between the GP, health visitor and a community paediatrician to see if any lessons can be learned from the case.

Using this risk factor approach, a cohort of 15% of babies in whom 50% of cot deaths occur can be identified.[3] This still means, however, that the other 50% cannot be predicted in this way.

## Does a high-risk approach work?

A 20-year analysis of the results of the Sheffield programme has reinforced the effectiveness of the scheme.[1] Babies born in Sheffield now have an average or below-average chance of cot death.

The authors' conclusions were, however, that the scheme was most effective in reducing cot death where there has been an abnormal reaction to trivial illness and where there is unrecognized serious illness. There is a tendency for families likely to suffer a cot death to be more mobile and to underuse or inappropriately use primary care services. It was found that the effect of the programme was to achieve a level of care in fact no greater than the average experienced by all Sheffield babies.

## What can the GP do to reduce cot death?

### Information

The GP and primary care team will be in contact with families during pregnancy and the neonatal period. The dangers of smoking and the importance of heat control, sleep position and identification of illness should be emphasized from an early stage. Indeed, the need to reduce smoking is important from the very beginning of the pregnancy.

### Accessibility

Illness in small babies is difficult to cope with even by the calmest of parents. For the smallest babies it is particularly difficult to assess the severity of the ailment. Most illnesses are trivial, but even so may produce alarming symptoms such as vomiting, pyrexia and inconsolable crying. There are also well-justified fears that there can be severe reactions to minor illness, and that tiny babies can become very ill very quickly.

Most GPs recognize the medical and social need to be more accessible to small children than would normally be the case. Worried parents need to be seen with the reasonable minimum of delay. Babies who are causing concern should be fitted in during or at the end of surgeries, however full they are. Reception staff should be encouraged to facilitate the early assessment of an ill baby. In some cases the health visitor may be able to see the baby more quickly and advise.

### High-risk babies

If the GP is aware because of pre-existing contacts with the baby or because a cot death scheme exists in the area that a particular baby is at especial risk, then accessibility and preparedness to visit are particularly important.

As far as management is concerned:

- The threshold for admission to hospital should be low.
- The need for early review should be appreciated.
- The health visitors should be made aware of what is happening.
- The GP should be particularly sensitive to clues that the carers may not be coping, and be sympathetic to this.

## What do you do after a cot death?

Guidelines have been suggested by the Foundation for the Study of Infant Deaths;[11]

1. Make early contact with the family to express sympathy and discuss what has happened.

2. Unless obviously otherwise, explain that a cot death has occurred, and that an autopsy will be necessary. Allow the parents to hold the baby if they wish.
3. Explain that the Coroner and hence the police will be involved, a statement will be needed, and that baby's bedding will be taken for examination.
4. Consider prescribing. Some parents or others may require short-term sedation, but most will understand that any relief can only be short-term and the work of grieving cannot be delayed for ever.
5. Consider suppression of lactation.
6. Consider the siblings. If there is a twin, he or she is at particular risk and may need admission for check-up. Other siblings should not be sent away.
7. Discuss the possible bereavement reaction. Anger may be directed at the GP, especially if the death followed a trivial illness which had been presented to the GP. This may make work with the family very difficult, and may require the GP to pass the case on to a colleague.

   The death of a child will generate powerful emotions, and some GPs will be unable to involve themselves because of their own unresolved feelings about what has happened. It is better for the GP in such cases to recognize his or her own problem and pass the case over to a colleague. On the other hand, a show of emotion from the GP can improve the relationship with the family and facilitate the open expression of grief by others.
8. Inform the family about FSID for written information and give details of their Helpline – 0171 235 1721.
9. Advise the company of a carer for the first 48 hours.
10. Make plans to see the family again when the autopsy results are available.
11. Offer an appointment with a paediatrician for the surviving siblings and for future pregnancies. In most parts of the country there is a paediatrician with special interest in cot death.
12. Ensure that there is good information exchange in any future pregnancies. 'Care of Next Infant' is a part of FSID and is available in many areas.

## What to do after a near-miss cot death

An alternative term for this is acute life-threatening event or ALTE. The at-risk groups for ALTE are the same as for cot death. The baby is found apparently dead and is resuscitated by parents or others. ALTE is more likely to occur in the day at a time when there is likely to be more supervision. This implies that if the baby had not been found, then death would have occurred.

The pathogenesis of cot death and ALTE is probably the same. All cases should be admitted, even if recovery is apparently complete. Very commonly an acute illness is present, and an important feature is that collapse is the first clinical manifestation.[12]

After discharge from hospital, close follow-up is needed. An apnoea alarm is usually provided. This is appreciated by the family, even though there is little evidence that its use will avoid a cot death. In addition, extra health visitor input is important, and this is particularly prized by parents.[3] This extra input is similar to the response appropriate for the siblings of a recent cot death.

# References

1. Taylor EM, Spencer NJ & Carpenter RG. Evaluation of attempted prevention of unexpected infant death in very high risk infants by planned health care. *Acta Paediatr* 1993; **82**: 83–6
2. Chief Medical Officer. Sleeping position in infants and the risk of cot death. PL/CMO(91)16. London: Department of Health. 1991
3. Taylor EM. Sudden infant death. *Pulse Ref* 1986; 31–6
4. Emery JL. Is sudden infant death syndrome a diagnosis? *Br Med J* 1989; **299**: 1240
5. Southall DP & Samuels MP. Reducing risks in the sudden infant death syndrome. *Br Med J* 1992; **304**; 265–6
6. *Back to Sleep. Reducing the Risk of Cot Death*. London: Department of Health. 1991
7. Report of the Chief Medical Officer's expert group on the sleeping position of infants and cot death. London: Department of Health. 1993
8. *Research Background for the Advice to Reduce the Risk of Cot Death*. Foundation for the Study of Infant Deaths. Factfile 2; December 1993
9. Thornton AJ, Morley SJ, Green TJ *et al.* Field trials of the Baby Check score card: mothers scoring their babies at home. *Arch Dis Child* 1991; **66**: 106–10
10. *Health Visitors' Confidential Report and One Month Survey*. Sheffield: Sheffield Health Authority
11. *Guidelines for GPs When Cot Death Occurs*. Foundation for the Study of Infant Deaths. London: 1992
12. Hardy JD. Near miss cot deaths: personal practice. *Maternal Child Health* 1991; 345–9

# Stress in doctors

## Aims

The trainee should:

- Be able to recognize any symptoms of stress in themselves.
- Know about stress avoidance strategies.
- Be aware of the need to maintain their own health.

## Is stress in doctors important?

The effects of stress in doctors are important for two reasons:

- The quality of patient care is compromised.
- The stressed doctor bears an extra burden of morbidity and mortality.

The effects on patient care are hard to quantify, but if most GPs are stressed most of the time, then 'normal care' will contain an element of suboptimal care because of stress.

The effects on doctors have been examined. GPs have more than their fair share of some illnesses, to which stress may contribute. Compared to the general population, GPs suffer:[1]

- Road accidents – twice average.
- Cirrhosis and suicide – three times average.
- First admission to psychiatric hospital – 2.5 times average.
- Drug addiction – 30 times average.

Emotional distress is highest in the early postgraduate years, and tends to get better with time. Work done on house-officer-grade doctors suggests that 50% are emotionally disturbed,[2] 28% clinically depressed[3] and 20% are regular or heavy alcohol drinkers.

The marriages that doctors contract tend to be longer but less satisfying than average.[3] Around half of doctors have had marital counselling, and a further 20% have considered it. Women doctors tend to blame lack of intimacy and time to talk for marital problems, whereas men blame the hours of work. Spending more time talking seems to improve the outlook for the marriage.

GPs tend to marry late, and typically have children quite quickly thereafter. Eighty-five per cent of married women GPs have children within 10 years of entering general practice.[3]

## Why are GPs at particular risk?

General practice has been characterized as a job with 'high demand and high decision latitude'.[4] This means that the workload is high, but this is compensated for by a high degree of freedom and autonomy in decision-making.

The 'high demand' part of the work has always been true. Recent surveys have shown that the workload is increasing, and that the changes that have been introduced since 1990 mean that GPs are increasingly being required to do jobs for which they are not trained.

The increasing regulation of general practice by government and by fear of litigation means that autonomy is being reduced. This makes the stress of a high workload harder to withstand.[4]

In one study,[5] 83% of GPs complained of periods of exhaustion, 68% found their work stressful, with 8% complaining of depression and another 50% of 'enduring boredom'.

Another larger study[4] found that, using indices of anxiety and depression, GPs were rather more emotionally unwell than their patients. There had been a worsening of the average GP's emotional health since the introduction of the 1990 changes.

Looking specifically at job satisfaction, 50% of GPs have seriously considered leaving general practice, and 75% regret having become a GP in the first place. Forty-five per cent feel general practice has failed to live up to their expectations of it.[6]

The work of a GP means that they may be particularly vulnerable to burn-out compared to hospital colleagues. They are always in the 'front line' of care, not cushioned by a phalanx of junior staff. The 24-hour commitment means that home and family life are disrupted at least from time to time.

Morale is also important. The chance of burn-out is related to perceived stress rather than actual stress.[7] If GPs as a group feel undervalued either by all the changes being imposed on them, or because their pay and status have not kept pace with other professional groups, then well-being is reduced and the chance of burn-out is higher.

## What do GPs find stressful?

The largest recent survey on what GPs find stressful[4] involved 1817 GPs in its first part in 1989, and 917 in the second part, completed after the introduction of the 1990 changes.

The items enquired about which correlated most closely with a low job satisfaction were:

- Demands of the job and patient expectations.
- Interference with family life.
- Constant interruptions at home and at work.
- Practice administration demands.

This work was repeated in 1990 to gauge the changes after the new contract. Measurements of depression, anxiety and somatic stress had all increased.

## How do people react to stress?

A certain amount of stress is stimulating and creates efficiency. The same stress affects different people in different ways, and the same person may react differently to the same stress at different times.[1]

Consider the relationship of arousal and performance:

1. At low arousal there is low performance, boredom – the 'drone zone'.
2. With increasing arousal, life starts to get interesting, to a state of optimal arousal when performance peaks. This is the 'C zone' of creative calm, and is the state to aim for. Life is busy but fulfilling, with talents being fully utilized.
3. By increasing arousal beyond this, performance begins to decline, inducing first fatigue, exhaustion, ill health, panic and eventually breakdown and burn-out.

## What is burn-out?

Burn-out is recognized in many professional groups, but there is no agreed definition. The term was first coined by Freudenburger in 1974[16] to apply to caring professions, but a similar phenomenon occurs in teachers and police.[8] It is unclear whether it represents a separate syndrome, or if it is just a variant of stress and job dissatisfaction.

Three independent but interrelated features occur:

1. *Emotional exhaustion.* Tiredness, somatic symptoms, irritability, accident prone, depression, excess alcohol use.
2. *Depersonalization.* Treating patients and others as objects.
3. *Low productivity*, and feeling of low achievement. Absenteeism, high sickness rates.

Doctors need to be alert to changes in their own feelings, behaviour and thinking.[7] There may be loss of sense of humour, a persisting sense of self-failure or self-blame, frequent anger or resentment, irritability at home and a progressively cynical attitude to patients.

Behavioural changes may include clumsiness and accident proneness, resistance towards patient contact and going to work, increasing professional and social isolation and working harder to achieve less.

Changes in thinking may include frequent thoughts about leaving the job, loss of creativity, poor concentration, unwillingness to listen to patients or colleagues, suspicion and mistrust of others.

Many GPs reading the above will recognize that it describes what they feel like, at least from time to time, and especially when under stress. It is probable that all doctors on occasion suffer some symptoms of burn-out.[7]

## What are the stages of burn-out?

Although stages of burn-out can be identified, they may not appear in pure form.[9] Some sufferers get stuck at one stage, others will jump from stage to stage at different times, and a few will follow a remorseless course so that all aspects of their professional and social functioning are impaired. They will also be very unhappy.

### Stage 1

This is especially common in the newly qualified, when starting work, or after a promotion. There is a feeling of uncertainty about coping with the demands of new pressures. There is a tendency to be over-conscientious or to overwork; in some there is a great deal of enthusiasm and energy. There may be guilt about personal adequacy, a compulsion to succeed, and a feeling of being trapped and powerless. The individual is unwilling to delegate.

## Stage 2

There are short-lived bouts of irritation, tiredness, anxiety and frustration. There may be feelings of stagnation or 'banging your head against a brick wall' plus a tendency to 'awfulize' – everything is awful.

## Stage 3

There is increasing anger and resentment, lasting for longer periods. There are feelings of failure and general discontent at work, accompanied by guilt, a lowering of self-esteem and feelings of inadequacy. Apathy and cynicism increase – 'Why bother?' The person is cynical, withdrawn, only doing the minimum of work; negative, rigid, unwilling to try new ideas, keen to crush enthusiam in others; and uncaring, unwilling to admit to personal needs.

## Stage 4

There is extreme personal distress. There may be physical complaints such as ulcers, headache and backache, angina, severe insomnia and other symptoms, with the abuse of coffee and alcohol. Extreme anxiety or panic leads to reluctance to go to work, depression or even suicidal feelings.

# Who gets burn-out?

There is an association between some character traits and burn-out. Some of these traits are particularly common among GPs and may have been the reason they wanted to go into general practice in the first place.

Of particular concern is the association of burn-out with doctors who are more patient-centred in their outlook.[10] The very characteristics which make a GP effective are also those which predispose to burn-out. It may be that those who do not burn-out are a group of 'survivors' who have succeeded because of an ability to detach themselves from their patients.

Personality traits commoner in sufferers from burn-out include:[1]

- Idealistic.
- Obsessional.
- Type A personality.
- Feelings of indispensability.
- Patient-centred.

A higher number of qualifications seems to be protective. Attendance at postgraduate meetings is associated with lower rates of burn-out, and is associated with GPs being less conscientious, more emotionally mature and more extrovert.

## How can you avoid burn-out?

The key is to recognize the possibility that it might occur. Doctors in general tend to regard themselves as immune to illness and stress, and to regard as a weakness any steps taken to reduce workload and emotional trauma.

All doctors have a professional responsibility to keep themselves fit to do their job to their best ability. An ill doctor will make poor decisions which may jeopardize patient care.

Since general practice is a 'good thing' in a moral sense, then there is always a 'moral' reason to do more work, be absent from friends and family, work long hours, miss sleep and not take holidays. As far as most jobs are concerned, this behaviour would be regarded as a dereliction of marital and parental duties. The families of GPs are torn between normal family needs and the assumption that when the GP parent is absent it's because there's something important to be done. The children of doctors have more than their share of psychiatric ill health.[11]

In the early stages, burn-out can be combated. However, it is evidently better to prevent burn-out before it starts. Being realistic about your own needs and capacities is an important preventive strategy.

### Choose the right job

- Be realistic about your consultation rate. GPs who are forced to work more rapidly than their natural style are more vulnerable to stress.[10]
- Make sure that how work is shared and decisions are made is fair, or at least fair enough to be tolerated.
- Are there likely to be any major financial worries? As well as personal responsibilities, this will also depend on remuneration and the costs of buying-in.
- Is the partnership stable or are there likely to be personality clashes or significant imminent changes in partners or other staff?
- Are there any extras – outside jobs, excessive on call, lots of evening meetings? Can you cope with sleep deprivation? It gets harder as you get older.

- How is out-of-hours cover arranged? Is there a deputizing service or local cooperative?
- Is the holiday and study leave allowance adequate? Is it expected that you will take the full entitlement?
- Is there local provision for postgraduate education, practitioners' groups or counselling?

## Organize practice life[12]

- *Managing paperwork.* Log the total amount of time spent on paperwork. Give paperwork the time it deserves. Give yourself quality time when you are mentally at your best in which to do the work uninterrupted. When you read something, act immediately: either file or throw away, and don't let it just pile up.
- *Writing letters.* Use a word processor to write letters, as this makes amendments easy. Or dictate letters on to a tape. Or dictate to a shorthand typist – it encourages accuracy. Don't type or hand-write letters if you can avoid it.
- *Delegating work.* Learn how to delegate. Do not simply unload your dirty jobs. Keep your nose out unless assistance is requested. Take a risk and give staff the chance: you will reap the benefits of working in a happier, more contented team. Staff need the autonomy and resources (training and equipment) to do the job. Make sure staff know when and how to ask for help. Persuade patients that others can do some jobs better than you can.
- *Organize yourself.* Recognize your weaknesses and act upon them. Make the most of your talents and experience. Personal efficiency is an attitude, not a rigid set of rules.
- *Keep the staff happy.* Don't annoy staff by giving them menial tasks to do all the time. Staff will be happiest when working to their full potential. It is worth risking a few mistakes. Keep the staff updated about what's happening in the practice so that they can remain an integral part of the practice team.

## Time management

### Types of problem-solvers
Traditional time management theory divides people into four types on the basis of how they cope with problems.[13]

- *Elephants* will proceed with their task to the exclusion of anything else, even if something more important comes up. The work is pursued ruthlessly and tenaciously, and they have no problem ignoring requests from others. Elephants are very good at taking the longer view and often find a role as planner. Tasks best suited to this approach are high-importance, low-urgency.

- *Monkeys* are geared towards achievement and are action-oriented. They thrive on high-urgency, high-importance tasks.
- *Butterflies* tend to be easily swayed by new ideas, and are easily bored and distracted. Staying power is not very good. Short time scales suit them best and they enjoy lots of variety and contact with people.
- *Ostriches* manage to avoid urgent and important tasks by spending all their time on irrelevant activity. This puts pressure on the organization and on other staff members. It is hard to see what useful purpose they might serve.

As well as these four groupings, some people work more effectively in the morning – the larks – and some better later in the day – the owls. Important jobs are best done when you are best able to do them.

Most people show a mixture of different problem-solving attributes, but with an emphasis on one member of the menagerie. It may be possible for an individual to alter to a degree, but any change will be difficult and slight. It is better to recognize what type of problem-solver you are and adjust the workload accordingly. When you are trying to work out where all the time disappears to, it is often instructive to spend a week writing down for each 15-minute slot exactly what you are doing. Later review of such a list can give valuable insight into what may be going wrong. Much of a GP's work is fixed by, for instance, surgeries and clinics, which may over-run for perfectly good reasons. Interruptions to attend to emergencies cannot be avoided. None the less, there will be slots of time in the week which can be organized to greatest effect.

*Principles of time management*[13]
1. *Prioritize tasks.* An urgent job is one which needs doing quickly. An important job is one which needs to be done properly. It is easy to leave the important in favour of the urgent, and if the important get avoided they tend to end up being urgent and so don't get the time they merit. Make sure you differentiate between urgent and important, and give jobs a priority level so that they can be tackled in the right order.
2. *Concentrate on your own tasks.* Many of the more stressful jobs are those which others ask us to do. Learning to delegate and say no is an important part of time management. As your talents rise

with experience, it is usual to take on more and more work. At first this is stimulating and flattering, and so you don't like to say no to a request. However, there is a limit to what anyone can do, and it's all too easy to exceed your capabilities or else take time from other important areas, such as relaxation and family time. Learning to say no is very difficult, but it has to be done.

3. *Time is a consumable commodity.* Once the 24 hours in a day have gone, they have gone. A job is worth the time allocated to it. When others want your time, there is a cost. The British Medical Association currently estimates that GP time is worth about £90 an hour.

These principles can be turned into a set of rules for time management:

- *Establish a routine.* If a surgery lasts for 3 hours, then do not try to rush and get finished in $2\frac{1}{2}$. A rushed consultation leaves you stressed and the patient dissatisfied, and any time saved is minimal. Make a schedule for other jobs and assign a time to them, and then try and keep to the schedule. Create time buffers in the schedule to catch up with yourself and, having established them, don't be tempted to fill them up again.
- *Work at the right time.* Important jobs require your fullest brainpower, and should be scheduled for uninterrupted times when you are freshest. Once begun, try and finish a piece of work, as if you break off it always takes time to 'warm up' again. Do not postpone unpleasant jobs as they will prey on your mind and reduce your ability to do other things.
- *Arrange uninterrupted time.* This can be particularly difficult in a job when emergencies may occur, but there should be some times in the week when you are not on call or otherwise committed. It should be possible to arrange with your partners at least one period without interruption, on the understanding that you will do the same for them. Important tasks can be scheduled for this time. The corollary is, of course, that there must be other times when you make it known that you are available to the staff.
- *Stay healthy.* Arrange breaks in the day when you will need a rest. The old idea of the tea break fulfils this end admirably. Say no to people if you cannot reasonably do what they are asking, or if someone else could do it better. Try not to take work home with you unless there is a good chance of getting it done: it is often better to stay at work to finish off and so leave relaxation and family time free for its intended purpose.

## How can you cope with stress?

All GPs feel stressed from time to time, and with many the feeling is permanent. The following can be used when you become conscious that stress is building up. However, it is more logical and sensible to accept the probability that you will feel stressed, and use these techniques in a prophylactic way.[1]

- Avoid self-medication with too much alcohol, coffee or tranquillizers. A third of doctors who come to be investigated by the General Medical Council have problems with drug or alcohol addiction.
- Work off stress by physical activity.
- Do not put off relaxing; use a stress reduction technique such as yoga, progressive muscular relaxation or a relaxation cassette.
- Get enough sleep and rest to recharge the batteries. Sleeping pills are unnecessary if lifestyle can be changed.
- If you become sick, don't try to carry on as if you were well. Seventy-five per cent of doctors admit to having worked when they were unwell.[9] Some doctors positively relish the fact that they have worked when unfit, as though it were an index of strength. Guilt and workload are the two most often cited reasons for such behaviour.
- Agree with somebody. Life should not be a constant battleground. Avoid entrenched interpersonal conflicts.
- Learn to accept what you cannot change. To ignore this leads to unhappiness, cynicism and bitterness. As a doctor you are overseeing a process of the ups and downs of your patients' lives. On the other hand, though they take up all your working time, you are only a bit player in their knowledge and experience. Friends, family and the television are a much more powerful health influence than the patient's GP.
- Manage your time better and delegate. The person doing a job should be the least well-paid person who is capable of doing it. Use a system that works for you, not against you.
- Know when you are tired and do something about it. It is difficult to go to sleep when feeling anxious or angry.
- Plan ahead. By saying no now you may prevent too much pressure building up in the future.

## What support can you get?

Doctors should be encouraged to give and expect support from their professional colleagues.[7] Postgraduate centres have a role in

setting up small educational groups. Stress management programmes produce significant short-term improvement in stress
scores. Training programmes can encourage self-awareness and
personal development. Training in specific problem areas, such as
administration, may enable the GP to cope more effectively with
troublesome aspects of the job.

Other support may come from within the partnership, or within
the family, though a sizeable proportion of GPs never discuss work
problems with their spouse.[11]

## How do you cope with a sick doctor?

About 95% of GPs are registered with a doctor, with about a third
being registered with one of their partners. However, in only about
half the instances when a GP consults a doctor is it with their
registered GP. There is a tendency for doctors to bypass their GP
and self-refer.[14]

Around 60% of GPs treat their own families, and over 80% have
prescribed antibiotics for themselves.[14] As there are clear advantages in the list system and the referral system, doctors are denying
themselves access to the best available care because of their actions.
In up to 10% of cases this misuse may lead to adverse clinical
outcomes.[14]

Many doctors have difficulty in complying with advice which they
would regularly give to patients. Doctors are particularly prone to
drug and alcohol abuse, depression and marital problems. These
are all areas where it is difficult to talk to a third party, especially
one whom you know professionally and possibly socially.

### Principles of care

- Do not self-medicate. 'The doctor who treats himself has a fool
  for a patient'.
- Do not refer yourself or your family for specialist advice without
  consulting your own GP.
- Do not prescribe or provide medication for your spouse or
  family.
- Do not attempt to diagnose your spouse's ailments or decide on
  the appropriate referral – leave this to your own GP.

If a doctor is suspected of being sick and not able to do the job
properly, this will often be noticed first by a partner or spouse.
Particularly with depression or substance abuse, there will be a

tendency for the doctor to soldier on and try and conceal the problem. The concerned person has three avenues to pursue.[15]

*Local Medical Committee*
In many (but not all) areas, the Local Medical Committee will operate a system whereby, if contacted about a GP, they will discuss the problem with the doctor's own GP, or seek the advice of a GP referee. This is a completely local system, and many sick doctors will be reluctant to have their problems assessed by close professional colleagues.

*General Medical Council*
If the General Medical Council receives notification of a doctor who may be ill, then the preliminary screener will decide whether fitness to practise may be impaired. Two medical advisers are appointed, and their reports are made available to the doctor concerned. Since the possible consequences of getting involved with the General Medical Council can be significant, a further effort has been made to set up an independent body to cope with the sick doctor.

*National Counselling Service for Sick Doctors*
This was set up in 1985. It aims to be non-coercive, and maintains complete confidentiality. There are 100 voluntary national advisers drawn from all branches of medicine and nominated by their royal colleges. The adviser will approach the doctor to offer help. If help is accepted, the adviser may take it on, or else call upon one of the 250 counsellors nominated by the Royal College of Psychiatrists.

# References

1. Kelly D. Professional burnout. *Update* 1992; **44**: 1163–70
2. Dillner L. 'Avoidable' pressures could relieve doctors' stress. *Br Med J* 1992; **304**: 1587
3. Hall A. Medical marriage: no bed of roses. *Br Med J* 1988; **296**: 152–3
4. Sutherland VJ & Cooper CL. Job stress, satisfaction, and mental health among general practitioners before and after introduction of new contract. *Br Med J* 1992; **304**: 1545–8
5. Morrice JKW. Job stress and burnout. *Br J Psychiatry Bull* 1984; 45
6. Cooper C. Young idealistic GPs are the most prone to stress. *GP* 1993; **8**: 45–46
7. Chambers R. Avoiding burnout in general practice. *Br J Gen Pract* 1993; **43**: 442–3
8. Mayou R. Burnout. *Br Med J* 1987; **295**: 284–5
9. Kelly D. Stress disorders: why are GPs such a high risk group? *Modern Med* 1989; 543–4

10. Moore P. Survive the stress of practice. *Monitor Weekly* 1994; **7**: 49–50
11. Myerson S. Under stress? *The Practitioner* 1990; **234**: 973–6
12. Lockley J. How to organise your practice life. *GP Newspaper* June 23 1989; 53–4
13. Brooks J. Time management. *Update* 1994; **48**: 406–10
14. Allibone A. Who treats the doctor? *The Practitioner* 1990; **234**: 984–7
15. Brandon S. Doctors who need help. *Med Monitor* 1991; **4**: 13
16. Freudenburger HJ. Staff burn-out. *Journal of Social Issues* 1984; **30**: 159–65

# Child abuse

## Aims

The trainee should:

- Have a high level of awareness for the possible diagnosis of child abuse.
- Know the local protocol to be adopted in child abuse cases.
- Be able to demonstrate appropriately professional attitudes when dealing with a case of child abuse.

## Some background

At 31 March 1991 there were around 50 000 children in England and Wales on Child Protection Registers.[1] This represents a 20-fold increase over 10 years.[2] New registrations were running at about 4% ahead of deregistrations.[1]

Four categories of abuse are recognized now:[3]

- Neglect.
- Physical injury.
- Sexual abuse.
- Emotional abuse.

Non-accidental injury (NAI) is a term covering all types of child abuse. Child sexual abuse (CSA) is often considered separately.

Before the Children Act 1989, there was a further category of grave concern, which has now been discontinued. Under the old categories, 50% of registrations were for grave concern, 15% for neglect, 25% for physical injury, 15% for sexual abuse and 10% for emotional abuse.[1] This adds up to more than 100 because some children are registered in more than one category.

## Physical injury

### What is it? A definition

> Actual or likely physical injury to a child, or failure to prevent physical
> injury (or suffering) to a child including deliberate poisoning,
> suffocation and Münchausen's syndrome by proxy.[3]

The term battered baby syndrome was coined by Kempe in the
USA in 1962. This described a problem known for some time, but
which had relatively recently become socially unacceptable. In 1880
Lord Shaftsbury, fresh from his success in improving conditions
for children at work, was none the less reluctant to introduce
legislation to protect children in the home, opining that it 'would
not, I think, be entertained in either House of Parliament'. It is not
that long since beating children at home and in schools was
completely acceptable to society.

### To whom does it happen?

Boys and girls are both abused. First-born children are more often
affected, and within a family it is common for just one of the
children to be abused and the others to be free from such abuse.
Young children are most at risk, partly because they are more
vulnerable and partly because they cannot seek help elsewhere.
Children under 2 years are at greatest risk.

Severe physical abuse has a prevalence of 1 per 1000 in children
under 4 years.[2] Death from abuse is rare after the age of 1, but there
is a minimum mortality of 1 in 10 000 children, or about 100 per
year in the UK.[2]

Much abuse is associated with angry outbursts, but in a minority
of cases the child is subjected to prolonged and systematic abuse
over a long period.

### In which families does it happen?

Most abuse is by the child's parents, and it is particularly common
for a parent or a cohabitee who is living in the home but not related
to the child to be the abuser.

Young parents are more likely to abuse than older ones. Abusing
parents do not usually have an identified mental illness, though they
may show personality traits predisposing to violent behaviour.
They may be unable to provide appropriate care for or control of
their children. There is also an association with unwillingness to
wait their turn to see the GP.[1]

Where a psychiatric disorder is present, it is likely to be a puerperal or other psychosis. Victims of drug or alcohol abuse are more likely to abuse their children, as are parents under stress through illness, bereavement or financial worries.[1]

Child abuse is more common in the socially deprived and in families without employment, but it occurs in all layers of society.

Abuse is calculated to be 20 times more likely if the parents were abused as children. On the other hand, more than a third of mothers who were abused as children provide good care for their children and do not abuse them.[2]

A priority for the GP must be to recognize the possibility that abuse has occurred, even if the family does not fit into the stereotype.

## How can you detect NAI?

There may a number of pointers to alert the GP that abuse has occurred.

1. There may be delay in seeking advice and treatment for an injury.
2. The reported circumstances of the injury may not match the observed facts.
3. Injuries in young children may not match what is possible bearing in mind the child's developmental maturity. For example, children under 1 rarely hurt themselves by running into things as they are usually unable to walk.
4. Watch the interaction between child and parent. The child may be anxious or distant. The parent may ignore the child's behaviour or distress. There may be known child-rearing problems, sleeping or feeding difficulties.
5. An older child may say something which gives a clue to the diagnosis.
6. There may be multiple small injuries in young children.
7. Disabled children are at extra risk of being abused.

## Which types of presentation are suspicious?

### Bruises

Bruises may be of different ages. They may occur on the face and round the mouth, and be caused by fingertips. There may be grip marks on the shoulders. Petechial haemorrhages can be associated with shaking, suffocation or strangling. Bruises to ears are unusual if not deliberately inflicted as the area is protected by the top of the skull and the shoulder tip – the so-called triangle of safety.

*Scratches*
Deliberately inflicted scratches are usually multiple and linear. The edges of hard objects inflict linear marks. All bite marks need careful examination as they also become readily infected.

*Mouth injuries*
Mouth injuries may be caused by blows to the mouth, or by forcing things into the mouth. A ruptured frenulum is a typical injury.

*Fractures*
Fractures may be multiple and of different ages. X-ray evidence may not appear until callus begins to form. Young children are at particular risk: one study showed that the victims of non-accidental fractures are under 3 in 58% of cases, and that this group sustained 94% of the fractures seen.[4]

*Burns*
Small round punched-out burns are particularly relevant as they can be caused by cigarettes.

*Scalds*
Accidental scalds are splash-shaped. Deliberate ones often show a glove or stocking distribution.

*Failure to thrive*
Failure to thrive may indicate any type of abuse. Particularly suspicious is the child who puts on weight as soon as admitted to hospital.

## What should you do?

*History*
The child may be presented by a parent, health visitor or social worker with either suspected or unsuspected abuse. The child needs to be seen promptly: some are in urgent danger, and in other cases an appointment delay may lead to the child being taken away without being seen.

A detailed history of the presenting problem and the explanations provided by all concerned is needed. It is not the GP's role to confront the abuser, but to secure the safety of the child and gather evidence.

*Examination*
The child should be undressed so that every part of the body can be

examined. Embarrassment may be spared to older children by replacing some clothing before moving on to the next area.

Examination should specifically include the scalp, ears, mouth and genitalia.

### Note-keeping
Case notes may later be used as evidence, so particular care is needed in their composition. Details of the history should include details of who said what by way of explanation of the injuries.

The clinical findings should be recorded as accurately as possible, including the site and size of any bruises and cuts. Diagrams can be very useful.

*If Abuse is probable,* then the child needs to be in a safe place. In practical terms this usually means admission to a paediatric ward. The vast majority of parents will agree with this. If they don't, then there are provisions within the Children Act.

*If abuse is possible,* records should be kept just as carefully. It is then recommended that the case be discussed with others more experienced, such as a paediatrician or a National Society for the Prevention of Cruelty to Children (NSPCC) worker.[3]

The NSPCC have a 24-hour hotline for professionals or members of the public with concerns – telephone 0800 800 500.

As a result of these discussions, it may be necessary to inform a social worker of your concern and let them deal with it. Social workers are the key workers in child abuse procedures, and should be involved at an early stage.

## Confidentiality

The Children Act makes clear what has been considered good practice for some time, namely that the rights of the child to protection outweigh all other considerations.

The General Medical Council, in its annual report of 1987, stated its position unequivocally:

> The Council's published guidance on professional confidence states that doctors may disclose confidential information to the police who are investigating a grave or very serious crime, provided always that they are prepared to justify their actions if called upon to do so .... On the recommendation of the Standards Committee, the Council in November 1987 expressed the view that, if a doctor has reason to believe that a child is being physically or sexually abused, not only is it permissible for the doctor to disclose information to a third party but it is a duty of the doctor to do so.

**What happens then?**

Each local authority area should have an area child protection committee which will set child abuse policy for the area. Such policy will vary from place to place, but will be consistent with the Children Act 1989.

In each case, after due assessment, a child protection conference will be convened. This will be attended by anyone who might be interested, including social worker, a health visitor, teacher, police and parents. GPs are urged to attend and contribute, and can claim a fee for doing so.

From this meeting, a key worker (always a social worker) will be identified, a care plan will be formulated, and a decision made whether to place the child's name on the child protection register. After this, child protection reviews will be called to assess progress.

The NSPCC is the only voluntary body in this country which has statutory powers under act of parliament. Through its 120 or so specialized facilities it can be approached for advice and to perform social worker-type functions.

# Münchausen's syndrome by proxy

The original Münchausen's syndrome was the term applied to people who fabricate illnesses and end up having unnecessary investigations and operations. In the proxy form, an adult (usually the mother) either claims symptoms for children, deliberately falsifies tests (e.g. by putting spots of blood in urine specimens), or harms the child, usually by poisoning or asphyxiation.

The prevalence is unknown, but is probably relatively low by comparison with all use. The first description by Meadow in 1977 reported 2 cases. By 1993, the same author had knowledge of 300 cases in the UK.[5]

The syndrome arises in the under 5s and usually starts when the child is 1–3 months old. Older children may actually come to collude in the deception. Mortality is around 9% of cases.[6] In 73% there is abuse of other sorts as well. The siblings of cases are also at risk: in one series 11% of the siblings had died in early life, 17% had been abused in other ways and 39% had suffered factitious illnesses.[7]

It is almost invariably the mothers who perpetrate this form of abuse. No one psychological diagnosis is responsible. Mothers are often failed nurses or other health professionals, married and of higher social status or more intelligent than their husband. They commonly become very friendly with the hospital staff where the child is admitted. The abuse may be due to attention-seeking, or an attempt to outwit the medical profession.[5]

In the typical case:

- The child's symptoms defy diagnosis despite being very dramatic.
- Symptoms occur only when there is nobody other than the mother there to witness them.
- Tests are invariably normal.
- The child's mother is uncommonly chummy with hospital staff, but won't leave the baby for an instant.

Management of Münchausen's by proxy is a task for the specialist. However, the GP may well be required to help pick up the pieces of the wrecked families that result from these cases.

## Child sexual abuse

### What is it? a definition

Actual or likely sexual exploitation of a child or adolescent. The child may be dependent and/or developmentally immature.[3]

or

The involvement of dependent developmentally immature children and adolescents in sexual activities that they do not fully comprehend, to which they are unable to give informed consent, and which violate social taboos or family roles[8]

### How common is it?

In the year to 31 March 1992 3800 children were added to child protection registers as having suffered CSA.[9] This is almost certainly an underestimate of the true prevalence. By tradition, 1 in 10 girls and 1 in 15 boys is subject to CSA at some time. These figures have been largely borne out by community surveys: MORI in 1988 found that 12% of women and 8% of men admitted to being sexually abused in childhood and 3% of women had experienced actual or attempted penetrative sex in childhood.[10] At a meeting of the Royal College of General Practitioners, 17% of the woman GPs and 9% of the males admitted to being victims of CSA.[11]

## To whom does it happen?

The following factors are statistically associated with CSA. The relationship is not necessarily causal:[11]

- Ever lived without natural father.
- Mother employed outside home.
- Poor relationship with parent.
- Parents in conflict.
- Stepfather families.
- Chronic physical or psychiatric illness in a parent.
- Parent sexually abused in childhood.
- Alcohol abuse by parent.
- Violence within the family.

## Who are the abusers?

About a third of sexual abuse victims have been abused by young people, mainly boys. Two-thirds are abused by adults: 95% by men and 5% by women. Most will have been abused within the family by a trusted adult.[9]

## What are the consequences of CSA?

Physical and psychological problems are much commoner in adults who have been sexually abused as children.

### Physical problems
Physical problems include pelvic pain, dyspareunia, menstrual disturbance, difficulties in childbirth, non-attendance for cervical screening, sexually transmitted diseases, frequent attendance with minor ailments. In one series 64% of women undergoing laparoscopy for pelvic pain had been sexually abused.[12]

Reluctance to be examined vaginally or have a smear is closely associated with CSA in childhood. This is a potentially serious problem, as 90% of women diagnosed as having cervical cancer have never had a smear.[13]

### Psychological problems
Thirty-three per cent of adult victims of CSA have psychological problems, compared with 14% of controls.[14] This rises to over 50% for those subjected to penetrative sex. The commonest diagnosis is depression, but low self-esteem, anxiety, obsessional neurosis, sexual problems, marital problems, parenting difficulties and eating disorders are also found.

## How do you detect CSA?

In 39% of cases the child reports the CSA. This is the most important indicator,[15] as most allegations are true. Some are malicious but it is commoner for children to withdraw allegations because they are put under pressure to do so, or because they fear the breakdown of their family. In 11% a carer or relative has suspicions. In only 18% of cases is the GP the one who suspects the diagnosis: GPs do not usually have a large role to play in the detection of CSA.[11]

The following features may suggest a diagnosis of CSA.[16]

- Aggressive behaviour, tantrums.
- Air of detachment – 'don't care'.
- Excessively compliant, watchful.
- Sexually explicit behaviour.
- Continual open masturbation, aggressive and inappropriate sex play.
- Happy only at school, kept away from school by parent.
- Does not join in school activities, few school friends.
- Does not trust adults, particularly those who are close.
- Unexplained abdominal pains.
- Eating problems.
- Disturbed sleep, nightmares.
- Running away from home, suicide attempts, self-inflicted wounds.
- Reverting to younger behaviour, depression, withdrawal.
- Secretive and excluding relations with adults.

## What should you do?

CSA is rarely an emergency in the sense that the child is at grave immediate risk of death.[17] In doubtful cases it is appropriate to discuss the case with a colleague, paediatrician or the NSPCC. The NSPCC helpline may be particularly useful.

The GP should be non-judgemental when dealing with possible abusers. They have a right to proper care just as does the child. Expressions of disgust are unprofessional and unhelpful.

When confronted with a possible case it is important to record what is said and by whom. Any examination should be cursory only, looking as much for other NAI as for signs of CSA. Most CSA victims do not have any physical signs – genital bruising and a torn hymen are features only of extreme abuse involving penetration.

If there is a suspicion of very recent abuse, then the child should be examined by somebody with forensic experience, which is more likely to be a police surgeon or a paediatrician rather than a GP. There is no justification in examining the child more than once.

When CSA has been confirmed, the same procedure as for physical abuse is activated.

## Neglect

Neglect is defined as:

> The persistent or severe neglect of a child, or the failure to protect a child from exposure to any kind of danger, including cold or starvation, or extreme failure to carry out important aspects of care, resulting in the significant impairment of the child's health or development, including non-organic failure to thrive.[3]

## Emotional abuse

Emotional abuse is defined as:

> Actual or likely severe adverse effect on the emotional and behavioural development of a child caused by persistent or severe emotional ill-treatment or rejection. All abuse involves some emotional ill-treatment. This category should be used where it is the main or sole form of abuse.[3]

## The Children Act 1989

Among its many other provisions, this legislation formalized the basis for the care of abuse victims and their families. It lays great emphasis on the importance of interdisciplinary cooperation and information-sharing.

There is also provision for using the Act to ensure the safety of an abuse victim:

- Section 44 gives a social worker power to obtain an Emergency Protection Order to remove a child to a place of safety. This lasts for 8 days with a subsequent possible extension for a further 7 days.
- Section 46 gives a police officer the power to remove a child to a safe place for 72 hours.
- Section 48 gives a police officer power of entry, by force if necessary.

# References

1. Price J. Non accidental injury in children: principles of GP management. *Update* 1992; **45**: 923–42
2. Meadow R. ABC of child abuse. Epidemiology. *Br Med J* 1989: **298**: 727–30
3. *Working Together Under the Children Act 1989.* DoH/DES. London: HMSO 1991
4. Price J. Nonaccidental injury in children: examination and diagnosis. *Update* 1992; **45**: 1003–17
5. Daniels A. How to recognise Munchausen's by proxy. *Monitor Weekly* 1993; **6**: 46–8
6. Enoch MD & Trethowan W. *Uncommon Psychiatric Syndromes.* 3rd edn. London: Butterworths. 1991
7. Samuels MP, McClaughlin W, Jacobson RR *et al.* Fourteen cases of imposed upper airways obstruction. *Arch Dis Child* 1992; **67**: 162–70
8. Schechter MD & Roberge L. Sexual exploitation. In: Helfer RE & Kempe CH (eds) *Child Abuse and Neglect: The Family and the Community.* Cambridge, MA: Ballinger. 1976
9. Bentovim A. Why do adults sexually abuse children? *Br Med J* 1993; **307**: 144–5
10. Markowe HLJ. The frequency of childhood sexual abuse in the UK. *Health Trends* 1988; **20**: 2
11. Wilson P & Furnivall J. Sexual abuse in childhood – a problem for life. *Med Monitor* 1990; **3**: 35–8
12. Harrop-Griffiths J, Katon W, Walker E *et al.* The association between chronic pelvic pain, psychiatric diagnosis and childhood sexual abuse. *Obstet Gynecol* 1988; **71**: 589–93
13. Wilson P & Furnivall J. Sexual abuse in childhood – a problem for life. Part 2. *Med Monitor* 1990; 302
14. Hooper PD. Psychological sequelae of sexual abuse in childhood. *Br J Gen Pract* 1990; **40**: 29–31
15. Robinson R. Physical signs of sexual abuse in children. *Br Med J* 1991; **302**; 863–4
16. Cloke C. When to suspect child abuse. *Br J Gen Pract* Connections (Suppl) 1992; **42**, VII
17. Roberts R. Child sexual abuse and the GP. *The Physician* 1988; 691–3
18. Annual Report of General Medical Council. London: GMC 1987

# 14

# Referrals

## Aims

The trainee should:

- Be able to list the reasons for making a referral.
- Be able to write an effective referral letter.
- Be aware of the issues raised by the referral process.

## Statistics

Overall 8 per 100 general practice consultations lead to a referral. There are large variations between GPs from under 1 to over 17 per 100. There is a fourfold difference in the referral rate between those GPs in the top fifth and those in the bottom fifth.[1]

Every year in the UK there are more than 60 million outpatient consultations. Of these, about a third are regarded as new cases. GPs refer most of these patients, though a sizeable proportion will have been internally referred within the hospital or from the casualty department.[2]

In 1986, the Department of Health and Social Security calculated that each outpatient attendance in a district general hospital cost £27. Dividing the number of consultations performed in general practice that year by the cost of the service gives a figure of £5.80 per consultation, or about a fifth of the cost of an outpatient consultation.[3]

## The history of the referral system

By the beginning of the 18th century, the physicians (whose Royal College was founded as long ago as 1518) had reconciled themselves to the emerging status of the surgeons. Both groups treated the rich who could meet their fees, and had complete control over the hospitals.

The less well-off were attended by the apothecaries, some of whom were members of the Royal College of Surgeons or held a licentiateship of the Society of Apothecaries. The apothecaries were threatening to gain status in the hospitals – a challenge which the physicians and surgeons wanted to fight off.

The Medical Acts of 1815 and 1858 tried to resolve this dispute, and to ensure the adequacy of medical training. This was achieved by the physicians and surgeons doing mainly private work, but having unpaid honorary appointments in the hospitals. The apothecaries were kept out of the hospitals, but their reward was that they became the only route through which the specialists could be consulted. The physicians and surgeons kept the hospitals, but the apothecaries kept the patients.[3]

## Does the referral system work?

The NHS achieves morbidity and mortality rates broadly similar to those in the USA at about 25% of the cost per person.

## Why does the referral system work?

Though born of interprofessional rivalry, the referral system has a compelling medical and political logic.

- Most patients are treated by the GP, which saves unnecessary referral.
- The GP retains a complete record of all medical contacts.
- Two different medical opinions are involved in the care of each patient.

### Clinical method

The methodology which GPs use leads to a low false-negative rate for illness, which means that they are good at finding the patients who are well.

Consultants use different methods which primarily concentrate on detecting illness. This methodology only works if the population they are seeing has a high prevalence of illness.[4]

The combination of GP and consultant methodologies is highly effective. To maintain this effectiveness the GP involvement has to come first.

## Exceptions

Exceptions to this logic are accident and emergency (A&E) departments where urgency prevails, and genitourinary medicine clinics which must adopt a wider population approach than the GP list can provide for services such as contact tracing.

In most western health services self-referral is the norm. Recently it has been argued that the absence of this facility in the UK constitutes a restrictive trade practice and an infringement of patients' rights.

On the other hand, patients in the UK do still self-refer to hospitals via (A&E) departments, having previously seen their GP for the same problem. In a 1992 study,[5] 20% of A&E attenders were sent by their GP, and another 10% referred themselves for a second opinion when presumably their GP did not feel such a further opinion to be necessary. This group of self-referrers had just as much chance of being admitted (around 30%) as other A&E attenders. However, it should be remembered that the doctors in most A&E departments use consultant rather than GP methodology when deciding on an admission.

# What are the reasons for referral

GPs are bound by their terms and conditions of service to refer patients on to other NHS services where appropriate. The reasons for which a referral to a specialist may be appropriate are:

- Diagnosis not known.
- Confirmation or exclusion of a serious diagnosis.
- Necessary tests or treatment only available in hospital.
- Second opinion requested by the patient.
- Sharing the load of a difficult case.

In a study in Oxford,[6] 35% of referrals were for diagnosis, 35% for treatment, 15% for management advice, 10% to share the load and 5% to reassure the patient or the GP.

# The referral letter

This is the usual form of first contact and has potential for much more than just booking an appointment. The information included by the GP may give valuable insights into the patient, family and social circumstances, as well as the clinical condition. Similarly, the consultant's reply can be an important educational device.

Hart and Marinker[7] have suggested that referral letters should include the following data:

- Clear identification of the patient.
- A succinct description of the patient's personality, but avoiding caricature and character assassination.
- A statement about the presenting problem.
- A summary of relevant past events, including treatments tried and the patient's response.
- The GP's formulation of the problem.
- The GP's and patient's expectations of the referral.
- What the patient has been told about the condition and the reason for the referral.

## How good are our letters?

The content of referral letters from GPs is not as good as it might be. A study of orthopaedic referrals in Nottingham[8] found that only the reason for referral, history of the problem and the examination findings could be found in more than 50% of the letters analysed.

In the same study, social history, family history and the information given to the patient (arguably areas where the GP should have more interest and knowledge than the consultant) all appeared in fewer than 25% of letters.

## How good are the replies?

GPs have shown a preference for letters about their patients which are structured in so far as they contain a problem list and a list of management proposals.[9] Around 90% of letters do not meet this preference.

The scope for education using referral letters and replies is also underused. Another study of orthopaedic referrals in Nottingham[10] showed that items of education appeared in 3% of referral letters from GPs. Educational content was found in 26% of replies, and these replies were more likely to be written by senior registrars rather than consultants or others.

## The referral debate

Referral is an expensive business, with each hospital attendance costing around five times as much as a GP consultation.[3] The wide variation in referral rate between GPs begs the question as to whether the higher referrers are wasting resources.

The referral rate of a GP seems to be an inherent quality and is not influenced by age, prescribing rate, experience in the referral specialty or practice size. Indeed, there is some evidence that experience in a specialty actually increases the referral rate to that specialty,[11] presumably because either the GP is more aware of what benefits consultant treatment may offer, or because significant disease is recognized at an earlier stage, or because as far as that specialty is concerned the GP is still in 'hospital mode'.

The only consistent features found in surveys which differentiate between low and high referrers are:[1]

• The ability to tolerate uncertainty.
• The desire not to look foolish to consultant colleagues.

It is not clear what the 'correct' referral rate is. There is a balance between conserving resources and ensuring that patients get the benefit of any interventions which will help.

Overall about 55% of referrals have a clear medical indication, but consultants accept the vast majority of referrals as appropriate[1] either because they appreciate the GP's dilemma, or because of the ability of their clinical methods to detect pathology rather than health.

A study of referrals to all specialties in one district health authority in the Midlands[12] found that 13% of referrals were inappropriate when independently assessed by specialists and a GP (between whom there was broad agreement).

The rate of referral is difficult to define. The number of referrals is easily counted, but the denominator to the equation is more elusive.

• Practice populations differ in age/sex distribution, morbidity patterns and social features.
• Within a group practice the patients registered with a particular GP are often very different from the ones she or he sees.
• Doctors within a group practice will have particular skills and preferences which will attract particular types of patient. It is sensible to look at whole practices rather than individual doctors.

## Is there scope for improvement?

The government not unreasonably finds the variation in referral rates between GPs disturbing from a financial point of view. GPs also have an interest in using resources in the most efficient way, but are rightly concerned that a reduction in the referral rate may lead to patients not receiving services from which they might benefit.

Two issues are raised.[11] By what means can the referral rate be altered? How can we assess whether all the patients who would benefit are being referred?

## Possible solutions

### Rationing

Rationing by charging the patient is a well-worn principle in most health services, but runs counter to the ethos of the British NHS. It might curb referrals, but there would probably have to be exemptions to the charge (in the same manner as 70% of prescriptions are dispensed to patients exempt from charges). Also referral decisions would have to take account of the patient's ability to pay rather than concentrate exclusively on the likely benefits of referral.

Giving GPs referral quotas takes no account of the lack of evidence that the differing referral rates of GPs are in any sense 'wrong'.

### Audit of referrals

Since the gaussian curve for the distribution of referral rates of GPs is so wide, it is impractical just to target the high referrers. The number of GPs involved in such an initiative would approximate to half of the total number.

Feedback on referrals, as long as it is ongoing, would be expected to make referrals more appropriate. This can be reinforced by the development of referral protocols between GPs and consultants to include not only clinical situations, but also the sort of preliminary work-up appropriate.

Under-referral is much harder to assess as by definition if a patient has not been referred you do not have a case to examine. One alternative is to use critical event analysis. When a problem arises with a patient, it can be subjected to analysis to find out if a referral would have helped.

### Fundholding

A central hope of fundholding was that it would make the GP–

hospital interface more market-oriented and hence more efficient. So far there is no evidence that referral rates among fundholders are falling.[13]

## References

1. Metcalfe DHH. Referrals: could we do better? *Update* 1991; 1093–6
2. Lydeard S. Improving out patient visits. *The Practitioner* 1992; **236**: 871–5
3. Marinker M. The referral system. *J R Coll Gen Pract* 1988; **38**: 487–91
4. Mathers N and Hodgkin P. The gatekeeper and the wizard: a fairy tale. *Br Med J* 1989; **298**: 172–3
5. Nguyen-Van-Tam JS and Baker DM. General practice and accident and emergency department care: does the patient know best? *Br Med J* 1992; **305**: 157–8
6. Coulter A, Noone A and Goldacre M. Why general practitioners refer patients to specialist out patient clinics. *Br Med J* 1989; **299**: 304–8
7. Hart JT and Marinker M. *An Exchange of Letters*, London: MSD Foundation. 1985
8. Pringle M. Referral letters – ensuring quality. *The Practitioner* 1991; **235**: 507–10
9. Rawal J, Barnett P and Lloyd BW. Use of structured letters to improve communication between hospital doctors and general practitioners. *Br Med J* 1993; **307**: 1044
10. Jacobs LGH and Pringle MA. Referral letters and replies from orthopaedic departments: opportunities missed. *Br Med J* 1990; **301**: 470–3
11. Marinker M, Wilkins D and Metcalfe DH. Referral to hospital: can we do better? *Br Med J* 1988; **297**: 461–4
12. Jenkins RM. Quality of general practitioner referrals to outpatient departments: assessment by specialists and a general practitioner. *Br J Gen Pract* 1993; **43**: 111–13
13. Illiffe S and Freudenstein U. Fundholding: from solution to problem. *Br Med J* 1994; **308**: 3–4

# 15

# An overview of geriatrics in general practice

## Aims

The trainee should:

- Know how to minimize disability in the patient with chronic multiple pathology.
- Be able to make or organize an assessment of function for an elderly patient.
- Understand the role of the extended team, and especially the role of lay carers.

## What is the social context?

### Changing age structure

People in the UK are living longer, the average age at death being about 72 for men and 78 for women.[1] The overall population numbers are slightly declining, the number of over-65s is stable, and the number of the over-85s is rising. In 1980 there were 500 000 people over 85 years. By 1990 this had doubled to 1 000 000.[2] This shift has two important implications for care of the elderly:

- The numbers of people in the normal carers' age group (women aged 45–60) is becoming relatively smaller. In 1900 there were 83 women in this age group for every 100 people over 65. By 1990 there were 45 per 100 elderly.[2]
- The proportion of economically active people in the community is falling. This is also exacerbated by the fall in the average retirement age. In 1960 there were 15 pensioners for every 100 workers. In 2025 there will be 30.[2]

### Health and social care

Each GP has on average 350 over-65s on the list. These generate 4.7 consultations each per year, of which 35% are home visits.[3] Ninety-five per cent of the elderly live in the community, and 60% are completely independent.[4] Thirty per cent live alone, and 40% with an aged spouse only. Two-thirds of the elderly are women.

Five per cent of people aged 65–69 have severe disabilities. This rises to 11% in the 75–79s, and 41% in the over-85s. In the first decade after retiring each person costs the NHS an average of four times more than a person of working age. By the second decade this has gone up to nine times.[2]

### Ageism

Getting older in this country is characterized by loss of status, declining energy, senility, ugliness and loneliness.[5] There is a sexual slant to this, as generally male status is defined in terms of career, and female status in terms of youth and attractiveness.

Eighty per cent of the elderly live independent lives; three-quarters of those who are over 85 can wash all over unaided, and 95% can go to the toilet. Ninety-five per cent of people over 75 do not have senile dementia.[5]

## Why is medicine in the elderly different?

Because of increasing numbers and increasing demand, the elderly are a progressively more important consideration for general practice. Their care is in many respects the same as for the population generally, but with a number of important differences:

1. The over-60 age group are reasonably tolerant of declining function. In one study symptoms such as hearing and visual loss, shortness of breath, loss of energy, joint pains and immobility were all regarded as a normal part of the ageing process.[6]
2. The elderly often have lots of health problems at once. In medicine it is generally considered good practice to try and tie all the presenting symptoms into a unifying diagnosis. This is often impossible with elderly patients.
3. Calls for attention for the elderly are often provoked not because of the effects of a specific illness, but because the patient's normal balance has been disturbed by what might otherwise be a relatively mild disease process. An episode of bronchitis in a patient who is struggling with dementia and immobility may require intensive hospital management, whereas such an episode in a patient without these other problems can usually be dealt with at home.

4. Most standard medical textbooks were written at a time when very few people survived to be elderly. Descriptions of disease processes relate to younger patients in whom presentations may be quite different. A typical example would be an acute confusional state brought on by a urinary tract infection. Such infections in younger patients are much less likely to result in global symptoms.
5. The elderly are more likely to live alone than any other age group, and so have less immediate family support. The maintenance of independence may stretch their functional and financial resources to the limit, so that even a small disturbance causes a rapid decline into dependence. It's no good doling out prescriptions if there's no one to take them to be dispensed.
6. The response of an elderly patient to medication will be modified by changes in physiological function, other disease processes and other medication. In general, the routes of drug elimination are less effective in the elderly, so that smaller doses should be used.
7. The well-being of the elderly patient depends more on care than on cure. Tertiary prevention, that is, the relief of the effects of illness, is the best that can be done in many cases. The aim of care should be to minimize symptoms and maximize function.

## What circumstances may cause a crisis?

When a crisis occurs with an elderly patient, there are usually one of four reasons for it – the so-called four Is.[4]

### Intellectual impairment

This may be brought on by acute illness, withdrawal of drugs, drug overdosage (prescribed or recreational) and sensory deprivation. Other factors such as pain and anxiety will distort intellectual function.

Underlying dementia may complicate the picture, or be revealed by the extra stress of the new illness.

### Instability

This may be due to cardiovascular problems, neurological illness and musculoskeletal disease. Drug overdosage or environmental problems may lead to falls.

## Immobility

Possibilities to bear in mind are musculoskeletal dysfunction, nail and foot problems, Parkinson's disease, mental illness and drug overdosage. Restraint by carers also reduces mobility.

## Incontinence

Urinary incontinence can be brought on by anxiety, depression, confusion and infection.

Faecal incontinence is most commonly due to faecal impaction with overflow. Other causes are tumours, colitis and rectal prolapse.

By the time the urgent attention of the GP is sought, the carers may be at the end of their tether and wanting to withdraw from care altogether. The admission to hospital required to buy some time may be considered 'social' by the admitting doctor. However, if it is suggested that such an admission is not appropriate, bear in mind that 30% of elderly patients admitted acutely to hospital die while in hospital.[4]

# What disease processes can mimic old age?

Though many elderly people themselves attribute a variety of symptoms to the inevitable process of getting old, it is inappropriate for the GP to reach this view without at least finding out if anything remediable is present. As some illness processes present differently in the elderly, and some processes are only common in the elderly patient, it is easy to become confused between pathology and old age.

There is ample evidence that in many situations elderly patients benefit as much as younger ones from intervention, particular examples being thrombolysis after myocardial infarction (MI), and the treatment of raised blood pressure. Also, as age is such a powerful risk factor for MI and stroke, the elderly have proportionately more to gain from the treatment of their hypertension.

Illness processes whose symptoms may mistakenly be confused with old age include the following:[7]

## Central nervous system

A common reason for deterioration in mental function is vascular disease. The possibility of cerebral emboli or arteriosclerotic dementia, transient arrhythmias and arteritis should be considered.

Alzheimer's disease is probably overdiagnosed and Parkinson's disease underdiagnosed. Neuropathy may present with loss of power and mobility, and may be due to diabetes, alcohol abuse or medication.

Depression, grief reactions and reduced sensory stimulation may all mimic dementia. It is not uncommon for more than one disorder of the central nervous system to be present, which makes accurate diagnosis more difficult.

### Musculoskeletal

Polymyalgia rheumatica is probably underdiagnosed, as is rheumatoid arthritis.

### Gastrointestinal

Poor diet, lack of teeth and malabsorption contribute to vitamin $B_{12}$ and thiamine deficiency and osteomalacia. The overuse of alcohol may lead to poor diet.

### Endocrine

Hypothyroidism is so prevalent in the elderly that some people advocate routine screening. However, a survey in general practice concluded that this would not be helpful.[8]

### Medication

Altered reactions to medication, and the interaction of different medications, both prescribed and otherwise, can lead to reduced function. This issue will be addressed later.

### Cardiovascular system

Atrial fibrillation reduces cardiac output by up to 40%. MI may be painless and present as confusion or falls.

## How can you assess mental function?

One of the most challenging tasks when dealing with a confused elderly patient is to assess mental function for dementia. A common type of dementia is due to cerebrovascular disease, and it ought to be possible to slow this process down. Other forms of dementia are in general terms incurable. With many forms of confusion there is at least a chance of improvement. In practical terms it is not uncommon to come across a patient with toxic confusion whose pre-existing dementia has made the confusion more prominent. Patients with poor cerebral reserve are more at risk from the mental effects of toxic disease processes.

The abbreviated mental test score[9] is a checklist which has been validated for use in the detection of dementia. Questions to ask the patient are:

- How old are you?
- What time is it – to the nearest hour?
- What is your address? This is for recall at the end of the test – the patient should repeat it to make sure it has been properly heard.
- What year is it?
- What place is this – name of institution or address?
- Can you recognize two people? For example, doctor and nurse.
- What are your day and month of birth?
- What was the year of the start of the First World War?
- What is the name of the present monarch?
- Can you count backwards from 20 to 1?

Interpreting the results:

- 4 or fewer answers correct – severe impairment.
- 5–6 answers correct – moderate impairment.
- 7–8 answers correct – mild impairment.
- 9–10 answers correct – no impairment.

## How can you assess physical functioning?

The Barthel ADL (activities of daily living) index is a reliable way of measuring physical and psychological functioning.[9] The emphasis is on the types of activity necessary in day-to-day life, and it does not attempt to identify specific disease processes. However, it is these abilities which make the difference between dependence and independence, with all that implies for the patient, carers and society.

Each area is scored on a three-point scale where 0 = no loss of function, 1 = some loss of function and 2 = complete loss of function.

- Bowel function (continent/occasional accident/incontinent).
- Bladder function – as for bowels.
- Grooming – personal hygiene, shaving.

- Toilet use – how much help is needed?
- Feeding – cutting up and eating normal food prepared by others.
- Transfer – from bed to chair and back.
- Mobility – around the house.
- Dressing – selecting and putting on clothes.
- Climbing stairs (able/only able with help/unable).
- Bathing – getting in and out, and washing.

## What are the risks of medication?

In the 9 years to 1985 the Department of Health prescribing data gave much insight into the pill-taking habits of the retired population (over 60 for women, over 65 for men). These prescriptions can be identified because they are exempt from prescription charges.

The data show that there was a 27% increase in prescribed items to the retired, the biggest increase (37%) being for cardiovascular drugs. An average of 2.8 drugs is prescribed per patient, and the elderly also buy 40% of over-the-counter drugs.

Some 30–40% of patients on regular drugs will have seen their doctor once or less in the previous 12 months. Twenty-eight per cent of drugs identified by patients are unknown to their GP, and 36% reported by the GP are unknown to the patient.[10] Compliance is no worse than would be expected with this confusion.

Age-related changes in pharmacokinetics and pharmacodynamics make the elderly at particular risk of side-effects. Some 10–20% of the elderly admitted to hospital have drug-induced illness.[7] The list of culprits is very long. All drugs causing confusion also increase the risk of falls.

In order to ensure compliance and minimize side-effects and interactions, the GP clearly has a responsibility to rationalize drug regimes for the elderly. Issues to consider include the following:

- Do not prescribe if the medicine is unlikely to help. Be ready to stop medication if it has ceased to serve any useful function. An example here would be the overuse of diuretics for peripheral oedema: they are unlikely to help oedema due to vascular causes, and can cause falls due to postural hypotension and hypokalaemia.
- Try and minimize the number of different medications being used. Combination products can be particularly useful here, once the correct dosage has been established using the individual drugs.

- Try and simplify treatment regimes. Once- or twice-daily regimes are likely to be followed, but with more doses than this, the chances of compliance are much reduced.
- Long-acting preparations, especially if they cause drowsiness, can lead to an accumulation of side-effects in elderly patients whose elimination systems (renal and hepatic) are failing. Longer-acting hypnotics such as nitrazepam are particular culprits. Dizziness is very common among the elderly, and many patients take phenothiazine derivatives as a result. As well as the possible dystonic reactions with these drugs, there is also the risk of drowsiness and instability.
- For confused patients, taking tablets accurately can be especially difficult. A regime can often be tailored to fit in with the availability of carers to administer the medication. Using special boxes may be helpful. In the Nomad system, a rack of small boxes is used, each representing a different time of day. These are loaded by the pharmacist with the correct tablets before being dispensed. The patient and carers can tell at a glance whether the day's medication has been used.

## Falls in the elderly

Fifty per cent of the over-80s will fall in a year, with a 2:1 preponderance of women over men.[11] In 10% of cases a significant injury results,[12] which is not surprising bearing in mind that this is an age group where osteoporosis is common. Twenty-five per cent of geriatric admissions follow falls, and they are associated with 4000 deaths per year in the UK.[11]

The number of falls is increasing faster than might be predicted from the ageing of the population. Currently 12% of the over-85s have suffered a fracture of the femoral neck, and by 2020 it is predicted that 25% will have suffered such an event.[11]

As well as physical harm, falls lead to loss of confidence and fear of falling. They constitute a common reason why elderly people elect to give up independent living and enter sheltered and residential care.[12]

### What causes falls?

Balance is maintained by a number of interrelated functions, the malfunction of any of which can lead to a fall:

- *Vision.* Only 22% of the over-75s are free of significant eye disease, commonly cataracts and macular degeneration.[11]

- *Vestibular mechanism.* Fifty per cent of the elderly have some degree of vestibular failure, though this can be compensated for if other balance modalities are intact.
- *Proprioception.* Input is received from the muscles and joints, especially from the neck and lower limbs. Arthritis can reduce or distort this input.
- *Central coordination.* Degeneration of the cerebellum and its connections becomes commoner with advancing age.

Each of these functions will tend to deteriorate with age, so that age itself is a risk factor for falls.

Pathological reasons for falls include:

1. Acute illness. Any acute illness can result in a fall.
2. Specific illness. Some diseases result in a high rate of falls:

   - Epilepsy.
   - Parkinson's disease.
   - Dementia.
   - Diabetes.
   - Carotid sinus syndrome.
   - Cardiac arrhythmias.
   - Stroke; cerebrovascular disease of all sorts.
   - Neuropathies and myopathies.

3. Drugs
   a. *Hypnotics.* Patients who have taken hypnotics in the previous 24 hours are at increased risk of falling.[12]
   b. *Drugs causing postural hypotension.* Postural hypotension is present in 30% of the over-65s, and it causes 5% of all falls in the elderly.[11] Diuretics, antihypertensives, antiparkinsonian drugs and antianginal medication are all culpable. Non-steroidal anti-inflammatory drugs may cause gastrointestinal bleeding which will lower blood pressure.
   c. *Drugs causing sedation.* Apart from the hypnotics, opiate analgesics, tricyclic antidepressants and major tranquillizers may all cause sedation and falls. In addition, it is estimated that 8% of falls in the elderly are due to alcohol overuse.[11]
   d. *Other drugs causing dizziness.* Non-steroidal anti-inflammatory agents may cause dizziness, benzodiazepines may give a sense of imbalance, and major tranquillizers and their derivatives such as prochlorperazine may cause parkinsonism and tardive dyskinesia.

4. Ageing. Changes in gait and posture, and the malfunctioning of one or more elements of the balancing apparatus can give rise to an increasing number of falls.
5. Environment. Like any other age group, the elderly can fall because of slips, trips and other accidents. However, it is not unusual for a particular fall to be partly due to the environment and partly due to deteriorating balance function.

### Can falls be prevented?

It can be argued that all accidents could be avoided as long as no one ever took any risks. For some elderly patients just living alone is a substantial risk. However, the institutionalization of all elderly people is unacceptable on psychological and financial grounds, as well as offending civil liberties.

*Ask about falls*
Having one fall is an important risk factor for having another. Falls may not be reported unless asked about.

*Identify the cause of a fall*
Identify the cause of a fall if possible. Environmental hazards are often amenable to remedy. Older people tend to live in older houses with steep stairs, poor floor coverings and outside toilets. A lifetime's accumulation of possessions may clutter passageways and make getting round the house more difficult. If there has been loss of consciousness causing the fall, then it is more likely that a fit or transient ischaemic attack is responsible for the fall. A witness account of the event can be helpful.

*Screen for risk factors*
Important risk factors predicting falls are:[12]

- Cognitive impairment.
- Muscle weakness, especially lower limb. Exercise programmes among the elderly will improve muscle power and balance, help stave off osteoporosis and keep the weight down – all factors which would be expected to make falls less common.
- Postural hypotension. Visual impairment.
- Balance and gait abnormalities.
- Foot problems.
- Medication.

*Take care when prescribing*
See earlier.
The psychological impact of a fall is often more damaging than the fall itself. Loss of confidence, fear of further falls, anxiety and depression can all follow a fall and produce dependence.


# How can the carers be supported?

There are 6 million informal carers in the UK, which is 14% of the entire population. Sixty per cent of carers are women, the usual age being 45–65 years. Twenty per cent of carers are restricted by their caring duties and half of all carers have long-standing health problems:[13] depression is particularly common.

The cost of providing such care through the normal channels would be enormous: Age Concern estimates that three-quarters of the £40b being spent on elderly care each year is provided by friends and relatives.[14]

Informal carers are hence a crucial part of how our society cares for its elderly citizens. In many cases the caring duties are onerous, and very small changes in circumstances can make the difference between soldiering on or going under.

The GP is often in the best position to assess when a caring situation may break down. Changes in the carer or the person being cared for are equally likely to precipitate a crisis when 'something must be done'. Signs of an imminent crisis include:

- Worsening of symptoms, particularly mental symptoms.
- Increasing contact with the primary care services.
- Increased contact of the carer with the primary care services.
- Carers will often tell you when they are getting to the end of their tether.

Within the family, care of the dependent member almost always falls most heavily on one person. This may be resented and give rise to family arguments. Occasional visitors to the dependent person may be left guilty by what they find, and one common response is to summon the GP, even though the situation may not have changed. Such visits often happen at weekends, and the call is frequently made by a relative who is not in a direct caring role and who lives a distance away. Such 'emergency' calls have been termed Jaguar visits since the Jaguar car is the typical mode of transport used to fulfil these family duties.

Carers can be supported by:[4]

1. *Communication*. Better liaison between service provision sectors, social services, health service and Family Health Services Authority.
2. *Information*, for instance medical information, details of carers' groups, available benefits.
3. *Making time*. Time for carers can be created by the use of sitters, respite care and day care. The GP can help by providing home visits, and by trying to see the patient promptly at surgery to minimize disruption for the carers.
4. *Simplified drug regimes*. See earlier.

## How big a problem is elderly abuse?

With so many carers under stress it is not surprising that occasionally frustration comes to the surface. The prevalence of abuse depends on definition, but in a group admitted for respite care, 45% of carers admitted some abuse: in 14% of cases it was physical. On the other hand, 18% of carers said they had been abused by their charge.[15]

A community survey of all over-65s reported that 5% had been verbally abused and 2% physically abused.[16]

Carers who abuse their elderly charges are more likely to:[17]

- Abuse alcohol.
- Have been abused by the dependant.
- Have higher scores for depression on the general health questionnaire.
- Have stopped work because of their caring duties.
- Be looking after dependants who are socially disturbed or with whom communication is difficult.

It is suggested that GPs and others should have a lower threshold of suspicion for elderly abuse. When abuse is detected, the priorities are:

1. Safety of the victim.
2. Physical and psychological health of the victim.
3. Physical and psychological health of the carer.
4. A plan to prevent recurrence of the abuse. This should involve the police, social services and professional medical colleagues.

# Is it worth screening the over-75s?

Research evidence from the 1960s raised concern that there was a lot of unmet medical need among the elderly. This conclusion has since been challenged, and it is now felt that the elderly are every bit as likely to draw their doctor's attention to their problems as any other age group.[18]

Attempts at disease-finding by screening have improved morale and mortality, but not morbidity. Most problems identified are related to continence, eyesight, hearing, teeth, feet, mobility, dementia and depression. The current view is that elderly screening should be directed towards functional assessment rather than illness.[18]

The 1990 GP contract[19] says:

> Under their terms of service GPs will be required to provide each year the following services for patients aged 75 and over. The services may be provided by the GP personally or by a practice team member. The capitation fee for these patients will be increased.

a. A home visit at least annually to see the home environment and to find out whether carers and relatives are available.
b. Social assessment (lifestyle, relationships).
c. Mobility assessment (walking, sitting, use of aids).
d. Mental assessment.
e. Assessment of the senses (hearing and vision).
f. Assessment of continence.
g. General functional assessment.
h. Review of medication.

In practical terms you can qualify for the increased capitation fee by offering in writing a consultation with the information that it can be done on a home visit. Between 66 and 93% of the over-75s see their GP at least once a year for other reasons anyway,[18] so the requirement for special visits is in fact quite limited.

This screening strategy is in accordance with the evidence in so far as it concentrates on functional issues. However, the evidence for vast unmet need is not convincing. One authoritative review of the evidence[18] concluded that improved elderly care was more likely to be secured by the creation of an environment where the elderly can express their problems, rather than by a rushed package of unproven activity. Another[20] suggested that the knowledge and training of the clinical professions were as yet insufficient to support a screening programme for the elderly.

# What other resources are available for the care of the elderly?

## Medical

All the population are eligible for registration with a GP (in fact, GP lists account for rather more than 100% of the population). Specialist or generalist services are provided by all hospitals. There is also provision for long-term care of the very dependent in a hospital setting.

Further hospital services are provided by day hospitals which have input from nurses, doctors, physiotherapists, occupational therapists, chiropodists and hairdressers.

There have also been experiments with NHS nursing homes. In the present climate tending towards the private sector for this sort of care, these experiments have been abandoned.

Community nurses are the mainstay of community medical services for the elderly. Their services are commissioned by the health authorities, except in fundholding practices, where the practice contracts directly with the nursing service. The nurses also have access to whatever night-sitting and bath service may be available.

## Local authority

The Community Care Act came fully into force in April 1993. This followed the recommendations of the Griffiths Report (1988)[29] to place the responsibility for care in the community on to local authorities. An assessment of the individual's needs is made by taking the views of expert assessors, and then care is planned accordingly.

Funding is provided by existing local authority funds supplemented by transfers from the Department of Social Security. By law, 85% of the money has to be spent in the private sector.

A key worker, invariably a social worker, is responsible for a care plan for each dependent person which has been agreed with all concerned. This plan should specify what services are to be provided and by whom. The local authority then buys care for its clients according to the care plan.

The philosophy behind the Community Care Act has been broadly welcomed by professional groups,[21] but reservations remain about its implementation, with 85% of GPs feeling that services are no better or worse than previously. These reservations are supported by charities working with the elderly who complain about the parsimonious attitude of some local authorities towards buying adequate services.[14]

There are now nationally around 5000 private nursing homes. Many of these opened during the late 1980s following the government's provision of Department of Social Security (DSS) funds to support residential care. The progressive reduction in funding levels from government has now left many of them financially vulnerable, and up to 30% may be facing receivership.[22]

Services provided direct by the local authority include:

*Home helps*
Home helps are available to help with housework, although in many cases their role has been limited in recent years. There may be a charge levied for the service.

*Wardens*
Wardens are employed to keep an eye on dependent people, either in their own homes or in sheltered accommodation.

Local authority homes (part III homes, after part III of the National Assistance Act 1958) provide permanent, respite and day care. They do not officially have nursing cover and are not supposed to have residents with chronic nursing needs, but most of them do.

*Day care*
This may be in part III homes, or at special day-care facilities. Places for the elderly mentally infirm (EMI) tend to be separate.

*Occupational therapy*
Community occupational therapy is mainly directed at providing ADLs and home adaptations, for which the council has a budget.

*Sheltered housing*
The local authority will have a number (but never enough) housing units suitable for the disabled, a group in which the elderly are by far the largest element. There is usually warden cover and suitable alarm systems.

**Voluntary sector**

*Age Concern*
Age Concern is a major national charity which sponsors a wide variety of work for the elderly. They provide drop-in centres and eating places. Literature is available for all aspects of growing

older, including services available, financial planning, support for carers.

### Luncheon clubs

These may be run by church groups or others, often supported financially from social services. For a nominal charge food, company and often transport are available. Some clubs are based on sheltered housing schemes.

### Meals on Wheels

Meals on Wheels service covers most of the country. The meals are usually provided from social service funds, and delivered by volunteers. There is a nominal charge.

### Pensioners' clubs

Pensioners' clubs are local self-help organizations with an emphasis on companionship.

### Transport schemes

Transport schemes may be available in some areas to help with trips to luncheon clubs, social events, trips to the doctor and hospital out-patients.

### Private sector

The private sector are integrally involved with the workings of the community care legislation. Those patients who are financially well-off will not qualify for state support, and may buy services direct from nursing homes, nursing agencies and others.

## How can you get hold of aids and adaptations?

### Hearing aids

Hearing loss is the norm in the elderly population. One-third of those over 70 and half of those over 80 would benefit from a hearing aid. Of these, about 25% have hearing aids, but a large proportion don't use them.[23]

Hearing loss is most accurately detected by audiogram, but an almost equally reliable assessment can be made by asking the patient, or by using a written questionnaire.[24]

In some areas it is only possible to get an NHS hearing aid after referral to an ear, nose and throat consultant, although in an increasing number of places it is possible by following a referral protocol to refer directly to the hearing aid department.

## Wheelchairs

Over 140 types of wheelchair are available through the NHS. There are 400 000 wheelchair users in the UK, half of whom are over 65 years old.[25]

There is a comprehensive application form which, when filled in, is forwarded to the local appliance centre. Community nurses, physiotherapists and occupational therapists usually have much more idea about wheelchairs than the average GP.

### Walking aids

Zimmer frames and walking sticks can be provided via the community nursing service. Sticks may also be bought privately.

A stick should be stiff enough to do the job it's needed for. The handle should reach the distal wrist crease so that the elbow is bent to 15° in use. A slightly longer stick can bear more weight, as the elbow at 30° can transmit most force.[26]

### Toilet aids

Toilet aids can be obtained via the community nurses. Examples include commodes, seat raises and bed pans/bottles.

## What benefits are available for the elderly?

GPs are obliged by their terms and conditions of service to advise patients of any benefits to which they may be entitled. This responsibility is usually discharged by having a few leaflets available, and by referring possible claimants to advice centres or social workers. Finding your way around the complications of benefit provision can be very difficult, which is perhaps why many people do not claim the benefits to which they are entitled.

A growing number of the elderly are as well-off after retirement as when working, mainly because of the loss of expenses related to work such as fares and insurance, and the lack of outstanding loans to be paid back.

However, poverty is a more familiar theme, with retired people three times more likely to live in poverty than those in work.[2] Two-thirds of all rent rebates go to pensioners, and only 4% of pensioners enjoy the same income as the average working household.

All people older than retiring age (65 for men and 60 for women) are eligible for free prescriptions. In some circumstances hearing aids, dental treatment, wigs and supports and sight tests are also free. The blind or partially sighted and those receiving a war pension can also apply for extra benefits.[27]

People on low income with little in the way of savings can get some relief with rent, council tax and heating bills. One-off expenses can be met with either loans or grants from the Social Fund. Details on all these benefits can be received from advice centres, direct from the DSS, or from booklet FB 32 available from the Benefits Agency of the DSS.

## Disability Living Allowance

The disability living allowance (DLA) is a tax-free benefit which does not interfere with other benefits.[28] There are two parts.

1. The care component has replaced the Attendance Allowance for those under 65 years old. There are three levels of benefit corresponding to the degree of disability. To qualify you must need 'frequent attention throughout the day in connection with your bodily functions' (where 'bodily functions' means things like eating, preparing meals, using the toilet, and 'throughout' means in the day as well as morning and evening). Alternatively, you can qualify if you need 'continual supervision throughout the day to avoid substantial danger to yourself or others'. Higher rates are qualified for if the care needs to go through the night as well. The disability must have been present for 6 months, except in the case of terminal illness.
2. The mobility component can only be applied for under 65, although benefit may be payable after 65. There must be difficulty with walking or getting about which has existed for 3 months and which is expected to continue for at least 6 more months.

## Attendance Allowance

The Attendance Allowance is a benefit for claimants over 65 years, as long as they are not already receiving the mobility component of the DLA, in which case they will continue with the care component of the DLA. The benefit is not taxed and does not affect other benefits. The criteria for eligibility are the same as for the care component of the DLA.

The DLA and attendance allowance are applied for using a standardized form which enquires only about the degree of disability. There is no medical examination required, but a GP or other signature is needed to confirm the presence of a pathological process, but not the extent of the disabilities. If benefit is refused, there is an appeals procedure through which a more detailed look at the claim, often involving independent medical evidence, is sought.

### Invalid care allowance

The invalid care allowance can be claimed by people of working age who are spending at least 35 hours a week caring for a dependant.

# References

1. OPCS quoted in Novum 49, 1991; 9
2. Questions of growing grey in prosperity. *Guardian* 1990; **22**: March 27
3. Glew C. Geriatrics Part 1. Next patient series. *GP* 1989; 25–30
4. Jenner G. Multiple pathology in the elderly. *The Practitioner* 1993; **237**: 119–24
5. Smith R. The church on aging. *Br Med J* 1990; **301**: 829–30
6. Fraser C. Patients' perceptions of symptoms in old age. *Geriatr Med* 1989; **19**: 49–50
7. Pelly M. Is it just my age, doctor? *Care Elderly* 1992; **4**: 340–3
8. Edwards Y & Davies TR. Usefulness of blood tests during screening of the elderly population in one practice. *Br J Gen Pract* 1991; **41**: 496–8
9. *Report of the Royal College of Physicians, London, and the British Geriatric Society. Standardised Assessment Scales for Elderly People.* London: Royal College of Physicians/British Geriatric Society. 1992
10. Elderly people: their medicines and their doctors. *Drug Ther Bull* 1990; **28**: 77–79
11. Lubel D. Falls and the older person. *Care Elderly* 1989; **1**: 66–7
12. Downton J. Prevention of falls. *Care Elderly* 1994; **6**: 24–6
13. *The Guardian* 1992; May 12
14. Tonks A. Community care fails the frail and old. *Br Med J* 1993; **307**: 1163
15. Homer AC & Guilleard C. Abuse of elderly people by their carers. *Br Med J* 1990; **301**: 359–62
16. Ogg J & Bennett G. Elder abuse in Britain. *Br Med J* 1992; **305**: 998–9
17. Pitt B. Abusing older people. *Br Med J* 1992; **305**: 968–9
18. Perkins ER. Screening elderly people: a review of the literature in the light of the new general practitioner contract. *Br J Gen Pract* 1991; **11**: 382–5
19. *Terms of Service for Doctors in General Practice* 1989. 1445/106. London: Department of Health. 1989
20. Harris A. Health checks for people over 75. 1992; *Br Med J* **305**: 599–600
21. Thompson A. Community care. GP guide. *GP Newspaper* June 10 1994; 81–2
22. Foster M. Nursing home owners lick their wounds. *Observer Business* 1994; **6**: 30 January
23. Hickish G. Hearing problems of elderly people. *Br Med J* 1989; **299**: 415–16
24. Sirimanna KS. Hearing loss in the elderly. *Update* 1993; 959–67
25. Young JB. Wheelchairs. *Br Med J* 1988; **296**: 625–6
26. Mulley GP. Walking sticks. *Br Med J* 1988; **296**: 475–6
27. *Benefits after Retirement.* FB 32. Benefits Agency of the Department of Social Security. Heywood, Lancashire: BA Publications. 1993
28. *Claiming Disability Benefits.* London: Help the Aged. 1992
29. Griffiths R. Community Care: agenda for action. A report from the Secretary of State for Social Services. London: HMSO. 1988

# 16

# Paediatric surveillance

## Aims

The trainee should:

- Understand the importance of a team approach to paediatric surveillance with particular reference to the role of parents and health visitors (HVs).
- Have the necessary skills to conduct an examination of an 8-week-old infant.
- Be able to describe a paediatric surveillance programme.

## How did it all start?

For many years there has been state provision for some groups of people to be examined for disease. An example would be the Contagious Diseases Act which allowed compulsory examination in garrison towns, and which was not repealed until 1886.

In 1906, the School Health Service was started under local authority control, followed in the 1920s by the Child Welfare Clinics, also under local authority control.[1] During this period infant mortality fell from about 150 per 1000 in 1897 to 70 per 1000 in 1922.[2] The emphasis was on 'provision of medical and especially hygiene advice'.

From this a series of regular medical checks of presumed normal children emerged, leading in 1967 to the Sheldon Report which suggested routine medicals, nutrition and hygiene advice, detection of defects, parental counselling, health education, immunization and vaccination, and the sale of welfare and proprietary foods as being the proper work of the child health service.[2]

The recommendations of the Sheldon Report were pursued without much question, despite there being little evidence that any good was being done. The observed progressive fall in infant mortality can be attributed almost entirely to improvements in living conditions and nutrition rather than to the efforts of doctors or screeners.[1]

A joint working party of the British Paediatric Association, Royal College of General Practitioners, the General Medical Services Committee of the British Medical Association, the Health Visitors' Association and the Royal College of Nursing produced a report in 1989 called *Health for all Children*, or the Hall Report.[2] This examined the available evidence and, with its revision in 1992,[3] informs the revised child health surveillance programme now in force throughout the UK.

## How are the terms defined?

### Surveillance

Surveillance is 'an ongoing process which includes a number of preventive and anticipatory measures going beyond the mere quest for disease. This is an integral part of the day-to-day contact that GPs have with children during surgery consultations and home visits'.[4]

### Screening

Screening is 'where a health professional initiates a contact with an apparently healthy child and applies a test in order to detect deviations from normality. Its purpose is the detection of mental and physical handicaps, defects of hearing and vision, behaviour disorders and neurological disability'.[4]

### Assessment

Assessment is 'a more specialized examination carried out because of suspected abnormality or the presence of risk factors, and is usually performed by those with additional skills in the examination of children'.[4]

### Primary prevention

Primary prevention is doing something to stop an illness happening, such as vaccination.

### Secondary prevention

Secondary prevention is stopping complications of an illness, such as treating raised blood pressure.

**Tertiary prevention**

Tertiary prevention is reducing the disability caused by a disease, such as physiotherapy following a stroke.

# Which paediatric screening tests are worth doing?

Serious problems in children come to light in four main ways:[1]

- Neonatal examination.
- Illness or injury requiring consultation with a paediatrician.
- Parental observation and concern.
- Detected by doctors or HVs in the course of a consultation for other reasons.

This is reflected in the three main emphases of the Hall Report:[2]

1. The content of screening should be determined by the current state of knowledge about the conditions sought, the effectiveness of the test and the availability of programmes for management.
2. There is good evidence that parents are far better than professionals at detecting a wide range of handicaps at an early stage.
3. The surveillance programme should include health education.

The only medical examinations of which there is strong proof of benefit are those for congenital dislocation of hip (CDH), congenital heart disease and undescended testis (UDT) in boys.[2]

Of the laboratory tests, only those for phenylketonuria (PKU) and hypothyroidism can be justified on the basis of the available evidence.[2]

The monitoring of growth is important, but there must be sufficient expertise in the various techniques of measurement to make it worthwhile. There is evidence that the necessary measuring skills are not universally available.

Hearing and vision are best determined by looking at the child's behaviour with respect to sound and visual stimulus. Looking at the eyes and a hearing distraction test are still recommended.

# Who should do the surveillance?

By tradition, doctors through routine medicals have performed most of the surveillance. This is expensive and unproductive, and fails to recognize the abilities of parents and HVs. Surveillance programmes should be led by HVs, with doctors playing only a 'bit part'.

The Hall Report recognizes the importance of parents to the surveillance process. Parent-held surveillance records are now virtually universal.

The aims of the national paediatric surveillance programme are:[3]

- To ensure that all children have the opportunity to realize their full potential in terms of good health, general well-being and development.
- To make sure that remediable disorders are identified and acted upon as early as possible.

## When is it best to do the checks?

A full summary can be found in the Hall Report and the subsequent working party report.[3] Only those parts needing GP involvement are given in detail. Although most of the checks are done by the HVs, GPs performing paediatric surveillance may be called upon if problems arise.

### At birth, or within the first 6 hours

This is usually the province of the hospital paediatrician, except for home deliveries and those in a hospital GP unit. A full general physical check is recommended, following the same pattern as the 6–8-week check. Tests for PKU and hypothyroidism can also be done at this time.

Health education advice may include nutrition, baby care, crying and sleep problems and safe car transport.

### First 2 weeks

Most GPs will do at least one postnatal visit, especially as it attracts a fee. A doctor or an appropriately trained nurse should check the hips again, but only if there has been no second examination before hospital discharge. This is because there are fears that testing for CDH too frequently can cause damage. This is certainly true in the rare cases of osteogenesis imperfecta.

Health education topics may include passive smoking, accidents – bathing, scalding, fires – immunization; reasons for doing tests for PKU and hypothyroidism; and haemoglobinopathies (when indicated).

**The 6–8-week check**

This is the check needing most GP involvement. It can usefully be combined with the postnatal examination of mother, or co-ordinated with the first vaccination.

- Check history, review growth and ask about parental concerns.
- Enquire specifically about concerns over hearing, vision and squint. This can be reinforced by the use of parental checklists. See later for details.
- Examine for weight, head circumference, CDH, red reflex. See later for details of the physical examination required.
- Confirm vaccination wishes, and deal with any problems evident at this stage.
- Keep the surveillance records up to date. This will vary with the type of record in use, but generally means making appropriate entries in the parent-held record.
- The Children Act 1989 requires professionals to act always in the best interests of the child. This may involve identifying some children as 'in need' under the terms of the act. Any such should be notified to the local authority as possibly eligible for additional social services such as care orders or fostering.

Health education topics may include immunization, dangers of falls, fires, overheating, scalding; recognition of illness in babies and what to do. These issues may be covered in the parent-held record.

**The 6–9-month check**

This is primarily the responsibility of the HV, provided that the essential items of the physical examination can be performed. Otherwise a joint GP/HV approach is required.

Parental observations and concerns are enquired about. Check hearing, UDT, CDH.

Health education issues include accident prevention, scalds and burns, falls, problems of increased mobility; nutrition, dental care, safety in cars; dangers of passive smoking and sunburn.

**The 18–24-month check**

This check does not require any specific screening procedures and is appropriately the province of the HV. If there are problems contacting the family, however, the GP should try and do the check opportunistically.

An assessment of gait and length or height is needed.

Health education topics should include: accidents (falls from heights, drowning, poisoning, road safety); nutrition, developmental needs, language, play, socializing; behavioural issues.

### Between 8 months and $4\frac{1}{2}$ years

The GP should check for heart abnormalities. This is usually just a matter of listening to the heart, unless a problem is suspected because of symptoms or unexpected clinical findings. In addition there should be a further check of testicular descent if this has not been done since 8 months.

It is appropriate to bear in mind the Education Acts of 1981 and 1988 which require that any child who may have special educational needs (around 20% of children) should be notified to the local authority at the earliest opportunity. This is a responsibility for anyone who might become aware of a possible need, not just the GP.

### The 54–66-month check – school entry

This check is done by the school health service staff. Height, and more detailed vision (Snellen) and hearing (sweep) tests are done.

Other checks or contacts may be required by local policy, for instance in Sheffield there is extra HV contact connected with the cot death and postnatal depression prevention programmes.

## The child health surveillance (CHS) fee

Since April 1990, GPs can claim a CHS fee for each child under 5 years on their list if they obey the rules, namely:

- The child must be registered with the doctor for CHS services.
- The surveillance programme performed must be in accord with local CHS policy.
- The doctor claiming the fee must be on the Family Health Services Authority's (FHSA's) CHS list. Methods of getting on to this list vary from place to place. In general, the GP should be able to show evidence of ability to do the checks, and must have the facilities appropriate for doing them. Details of how to get on to the local list can be obtained from the FHSA. Being on one FHSA's list does not automatically qualify you for admission to another's.

The CHS fee is currently £10.50 per child,[5] or about a quarter of the fee for a completed course of infant vaccinations.

The GP contract is quite vague. You are required to do (or have done on your behalf) such examinations as are deemed fit by 'the relevant health authority', and to keep adequate records of what has been done and found.[6] The power is thus all in the hands of the district health authority (DHA) and its agents.

As an example, the requirements to be on the Sheffield CHS list are to have proved to the DHA that you have had either experience in child surveillance or recent hospital training, and have attended a course on local CHS policy which lasts about 2 hours. CHS clinics are to be held on a specified half-day each week, and not at the same time as ill patients are being seen. HVs should be in attendance, and there should be sufficient regard for safety. The local version of the parent-held record should be used to record what has happened. The CHS clinical policy which it is necessary to follow is detailed in a joint FHSA/DHA document, and this sets out what should be done when and by whom.

## How can congenital dislocation of the hip be detected?

CDH is defined as: 'a congenital deformation of the hip joint in which the head of the femur is (or may be) partially or completely displaced from the acetabulum'.[7] It thus includes instability, subluxation and dysplasia, so the term dislocation is misleading.

At birth 15–20 per 1000 babies have evidence of hip instability, but in 60% of cases the signs resolve in the first week of life without treatment. However, 10% of unstable hips will persist to show classic signs of dislocation in later infant life, and another 10% will later show evidence of dysplasia and/or subluxation.[7]

The tests used to detect CHD are not particularly good. Children have to be tested several times, and you can only be sure that a hip is normal when the child is walking with a normal gait.

### At-risk groups

Most cases of CHD occur in girls and in first-born babies. In 60% of cases of CHD, the following risk factors can be found:

- Family history of CHD.
- Breech delivery.
- Other congenital postural deformity, e.g. foot problems.
- Caesarean section delivery.
- Oligohydramnios or fetal growth retardation.

**When to screen**

It is recommended that tests be done within 24 hours of birth, before hospital discharge or within the first 2 weeks of life, at 6 weeks, between 6 and 9 months and between 15 and 21 months. In addition, gait should be reviewed at $2\frac{1}{2}$ years.

**How to test**

A total of 80–90% of cases can be identified by trained and committed workers. After the age of 6 weeks as the legs extend, the classical signs of CDH become more common. Bilateral CDH is harder to spot than unilateral CDH because there is no normal hip for comparison.

*Classical signs*
- Leg posture: partial lateral rotation, flexion and abduction.
- Limb shortening: above-knee shortening on the affected side.
- Asymmetry of thighs: skin creases observed from the front.
- Flattening of the buttock.
- Limitation of abduction: a normal hip in flexion should abduct more than 75°.
- Hip instability: specific testing may reveal movement of the femoral head in and out of the acetabulum. Clicking in the absence of movement (or 'clunk') is ligamentous and of no significance.

*Gait*
Most CHD cases walk at the normal time. However, at 18 months 20% are not walking, compared to the normal 5%. Any child not walking at 18 months should be tested for CDH.

*Trendelenburg's sign*
At any age over 2 years, ask the child to stand on one leg. When standing on a leg with CDH, the hip abductors have no fulcrum to hold the pelvis level. This is compensated for by the child leaning over to the affected side – the so-called Trendelenburg-positive.

*Ortolani test*
The child is laid on his back with the hip flexed to a right angle and the knees flexed. Starting with the knees together the hips are slowly abducted, and if one is dislocated, somewhere in the 90° arc of abduction the femur slips (forward) back into the acetabulum with a visible and palpable jerk.[8]

*Barlow test part 1*

The child is laid on his back. The hips are flexed in a right angle and the knees are fully flexed. The middle finger of each hand is closed over the greater trochanter and the thumb of each hand is applied to the inner side of the thigh close but not quite in the groin. The hips are carried into abduction. With the hips at about 70° of abduction the middle finger of each hand in turn exerts pressure away from the examining couch as if to push the trochanter towards the symphysis pubis. In a normal child no movement occurs. If the hip is dislocated, the greater trochanter and the head of the femur with it can be felt to move in the direction in which the pressure has been applied.[8]

*Barlow test part 2*

With the hip in the same position as described, the thumb, which is applied over the upper not inner part of the thigh, exerts pressure towards the couch. In a normal child no movement occurs. In a child with CDH the head of the femur can be felt to slip out and come back immediately the pressure is released.[8]

After the first month the most important test is limited abduction of the hip when fully flexed.

If on testing it is suspected that the child has CHD (which includes a subluxable hip), then there should be a referral to a hospital colleague. Tests from a more experienced hand and access to ultrasound imaging will throw more light on the case.

## How can congenital heart disease be detected?

Congenital heart disease is a fairly common defect arising in 6 per 1000 births, but each GP will only see 1 every 5 years.[9] Most present soon after birth, but atrial septal defect (ASD) and pulmonary stenosis (PS) may not present till childhood. A later heart check at 8–54 months is recommended.

Minor degrees of ventricular septal defect, ASD or PS, while not serious, still require anti-endocarditis prophylaxis.

Innocent murmurs are common up to age 12 years, especially in febrile children. The murmur is soft (less than 3/6), localized to the left sternal edge and always systolic. Heart sounds are normal and there are no other symptoms or signs of heart disease.

Pathological murmurs are usually louder than 3/6, may radiate and may be systolic or diastolic. Heart sounds may be abnormal, and other symptoms of heart disease may be present such as tachypnoea, poor feeding and weight gain, abnormal blood pressure, loss of peripheral pulses, a palpable thrill, cyanosis or evidence of congestive cardiac failure such as an enlarged liver or basal chest crepitations.

## How can undescended testis be detected?

Six per cent of boys are born with one or both testes not in the scrotum. By 3 months only 1.6% remain undescended, and few testes descend after 6 months. Very rarely, previously descended testes may ascend. Delayed descent may lead to subfertility, and there is a 5% chance of malignant change in the UDT.[10]

If UDT is detected at the 8-week check, it can either be rechecked at 3 months or else referred straight on to the surgeons. If surgery is needed it should be done around the first birthday. The presence of a hernia makes surgery more likely.

Cold hands and too much vigour make testes retract.

## How can development be assessed?

It is now recommended that most of the routine developmental checks are done by the HV staff.[3] If a problem is suspected, then the GP will become involved for a second opinion. HVs are highly trained workers and their opinions should be taken seriously. If they think there is a problem, they are usually correct. A specialist referral will usually be required.

A team approach to CHS requires that the autonomy and skills of each worker are respected. Having proper regard to the opinions of HVs is important to this end. The authority and competence of the HV are also reinforced as far as the child's parents are concerned.

- At 8 weeks most babies will be smiling, making noises other than crying, and fixing on and following mother's face.
- With the trunk supported, there should be good head control.
- In ventral suspension, the arms and legs should be flexed and the head should be held horizontal, at least for short periods.

## How can vision be assessed?

At 8 weeks it's not worth checking vision, but a red reflex should be looked for, as should evidence of squint. Divergent squint is always abnormal. Convergent squint may be observed for a few months if everything else is all right.

Parental observation is the most reliable way of detecting abnormality.[9] Checklists are available to help the parents' assessment:

- Does your baby look at you, follow your face and smile back?
- Do the baby's eyes move together?
- Do you think a squint is developing?
- Does your baby turn towards light?

## How can hearing problems be detected?

Once more, parental observation is the best way of detecting any problems. Specific questions can be used:[9]

- Is your baby startled by sudden loud noises (such as a hand clap or slammed door)? A normal reaction is for the baby to blink and open the eyes.
- Are prolonged sounds being noticed? The baby should pause and listen when, for instance, a vacuum cleaner is turned on.

While a routine hearing test is not helpful, the at-risk status of the baby may lead to referral for more detailed testing. The at-risk group includes:

- Family history of childhood deafness.
- Congenital abnormalities present, especially craniofacial.
- Chromosomal abnormalities, especially Down's.
- Neonatal asphyxia.
- Ventricular haemorrhage.
- Maternal infections: *cytomegalovirus*, rubella, *Toxoplasma*.
- Birth weight under 1.5 kg.

## References

1. Hannay D. *Future of General Practice and Child Health*. Sheffield: Sheffield University. 1989
2. Polnay L and Hall DMB. Child health surveillance. *Br Med J* 1989; **299**: 1351–3
3. *Report of the Second Joint Working Party on Child Health Surveillance (1990)*. Chair: Waine C. PL/CMO (92) 3. London: Department of Health. 1992
4. Bain J. Developmental screening for pre-school children: is it worthwhile? *J R Coll Gen Pract* 1989; **39**: 133–7

5. Database. Medeconomics, **15**, September 1994
6. *National Health Service (General Medical Services) Regulations.* London: HMSO. 1992
7. *Screening for the Detection of Congenital Dislocation of the Hip.* London: Standing Medical Advisory Committee. 1986
8. Sharrard W. In: The Newborn. *Pulse,* **44**, June 1994
9. *Clinical Policy for Child Health Surveillance and Immunisation (Preschool),* 2nd edn. Sheffield: Sheffield Health Authority and Sheffield FHSA. 1993
10. *The Examination of the Testes in Childhood.* Sheffield: Sheffield FHSA/DHA. 1989

# Index